THE ADHD RECIPE BOOK

Tips, planners and 90 easy recipes to eat well with ADHD

JACQUELINE GALANTY

hamlyn

hamlyn

First published in Great Britain in 2026 by Hamlyn,
an imprint of Octopus Publishing Group Ltd
Carmelite House
50 Victoria Embankment
London EC4Y 0DZ
www.octopusbooks.co.uk

An Hachette UK Company
www.hachette.co.uk

The authorized representative in the EEA is Hachette Ireland, 8 Castlecourt Centre, Dublin 15, D15 XTP3, Ireland (email: info@hbgi.ie)

Some of this material previously appeared in *HAC 200 Easy Cakes & Bakes, HAC 200 Easy Vegetarian Dishes, HAC 200 Fast Family Favourites, HAC 200 Gluten-Free Recipes, HAC 200 Low Calorie Recipes, HAC 200 Low Fat Dishes, HAC 200 Meals for Two, HAC 200 Mexican Dishes, HAC 200 More One Pot Meals, HAC 200 One Pot Meals, HAC 200 Pasta Dishes, HAC 200 Really Easy Recipes, HAC 200 Recipes for Kids, HAC 200 Super Salads, HAC 200 Tapas & Spanish Dishes, HAC 200 Ten-Minute Meals, HAC 200 Twenty-Minute Meals, HAC 200 Vegan Recipes, HAC 200 Veggie Feasts, HQC Budget, HQC Cakes & Bakes, HQC Desserts, HQC Fish, HQC Gluten Free, HQC Healthy Feasts, HQC Italian, HQC Low Fat, HQC Midweek Meals, HQC Moroccan, HQC One Pot, HQC Pasta, HQC Student, HQC Vegetarian* and *HQC Winter Warmers*.

Distributed in the US by Hachette Book Group, 1290 Avenue of the Americas, 4th and 5th Floors, New York, NY 10104

Distributed in Canada by Canadian Manda Group, 664 Annette St., Toronto, Ontario, Canada M6S 2C8

ISBN: 978-0-600-64026-4
eISBN: 978-0-600-64028-8

MIX
Paper | Supporting responsible forestry
FSC® C008047

A CIP catalogue record for this book is available from the British Library.

Printed and bound in China.

10 9 8 7 6 5 4 3 2 1

Commissioned by: Alice Gawthrop
Art Director: Jaz Bahra
Editor: Scarlet Furness
Copy Editor: Vicky Orchard
Production Managers: Lucy Carter and Nic Jones

Standard level spoon measurements are used in all recipes.
1 tablespoon = one 15 ml spoon
1 teaspoon = one 5 ml spoon

Both imperial and metric measurements have been given in all recipes. Use one set of measurements only and not a mixture of both.

Eggs should be medium unless otherwise stated. The Department of Health advises that eggs should not be consumed raw. This book contains dishes made with raw or lightly cooked eggs. It is prudent for more vulnerable people such as pregnant and nursing mothers, the elderly, babies and young children to avoid uncooked or lightly cooked dishes made with eggs. Once prepared these dishes should be kept refrigerated and used promptly.

Milk should be full fat unless otherwise stated.

Fresh herbs should be used unless otherwise stated. If unavailable use dried herbs as an alternative but halve the quantities stated.

Ovens should be preheated to the specific temperature – if using a fan-assisted oven, follow manufacturer's instructions for adjusting the time and the temperature.

All microwave information is based on a 700-watt oven. Follow manufacturer's instructions for an oven with a different wattage.

Pepper should be freshly ground black pepper unless otherwise stated.

This book includes dishes made with nuts and nut derivatives. It is advisable for customers with known allergic reactions to nuts and nut derivatives and those who may be potentially vulnerable to these allergies, such as babies and children with a family history of allergies, to avoid dishes made with nuts and nut oils. It is also prudent to check the labels of pre-prepared ingredients for the possible inclusion of nut derivatives.

Vegetarians should look for the 'V' symbol on a cheese to ensure it is made with vegetarian rennet.

Contents

What is ADHD?

In my work as a dietitian, I work with many clients who have recently been diagnosed with **attention deficit hyperactivity disorder (ADHD)**. Often, they arrive at my door because they've just made the connection between ADHD and the way they eat.

To better understand this relationship, it can be useful to start with understanding how ADHD can affect your behaviour across different parts of life.

Recognizing and understanding ADHD can help you to work out how it affects your everyday routines like eating and self-care. When you understand it, you can organize your life to channel the advantages of ADHD and manage its challenges.

Descriptions of ADHD focus on the traits used for diagnosis – impulsivity, inattention and hyperactivity.

- You may notice **impulsivity** as the tendency to jump in before you've had time to think things through. This might mean blurting something out, taking a risk or acting on a gut feeling.
- **Inattention** is when it's difficult to stay focused without getting distracted by everything going on around you or struggling to finish what you've started.
- **Hyperactivity** is having energy and feeling like you are always on the go, whether it's moving, talking or simply feeling restless inside.

Most people have a mix of these traits, and that blend is different for everyone.

Everyone loses focus or acts on impulse sometimes. ADHD is when these patterns are strong, persistent and show up across different parts of life – at home, at work or school. Crucially, they can get in the way of day to day living. That's the 'disorder' part of ADHD.

It's possible to set up your environment to limit the negative effects of these traits and channel their advantages:

- **Impulsivity** in the right time and place can be **spontaneity**, or the ability to seize the moment and bring energy or creativity into situations.
- The flip side of **inattention** is **perceptiveness** – maybe you notice details, patterns or emotions that others often miss.
- **Hyperactivity** in a less confined situation is simply being '**active**' or having the drive, stamina and enthusiasm to keep moving things forward.

Population surveys show approximately 4% of children and 3% of adults meet the criteria for ADHD, yet diagnosis rates are at about 1% in the UK, suggesting that it's often missed. That said, ADHD is becoming more understood and accepted and awareness in schools, healthcare and workplaces is improving. This makes it easier to recognize the symptoms and access support.

For example, we now have a better understanding that ADHD often presents differently in girls and has historically gone under-diagnosed. There is also greater awareness that it often continues into adulthood, with more adults getting diagnosed and supported.

Many of my clients approach me because they find that their experience of ADHD shapes the way they eat in their daily lives. Sometimes it's not a formal diagnosis at all, but little signs that ADHD might be quietly getting in the way of planning meals, sticking to routines, staying organized.

Once we start talking about food, the conversation often opens up into other parts of life too.

Eating Well for Health & ADHD

Eating well lays the foundation for your health. It **fuels your body, steadies your mood**, **supports focus** and **sharpens memory**. When you're nourished:

- sleep comes more easily
- stress feels more manageable
- your energy is steadier across the day.

In the long term, balanced eating lowers the risk of illness and supports wellbeing.

This sounds simple but modern life is busy and complicated, and this can get in the way of our best intentions. Stress, poor sleep and busy schedules can push eating off course.

Sometimes, this means turning to convenience foods or eating larger amounts than usual when we're tired and need comfort. Other times, it's the opposite and the same pressures mean we lose our appetite, skip meals or find food preparation too exhausting to even start.

Add to that the constant availability of eating out options, persuasive advertising and a culture that celebrates dieting and meal skipping, and it's no surprise that eating well feels hard.

For people living with ADHD, these challenges are magnified. Research shows that people with ADHD eat fewer fruits, vegetables and protein-rich foods, and more processed options than the general population. This is partly because **eating well depends on a hidden set of skills, and ADHD can make some of these harder**. Some of the common barriers can be found in the table opposite.

This recipe book is more than a collection of meals – it's designed to work with an ADHD brain. The food is nourishing and the recipes are structured simply with realistic planning tips to take the friction out of cooking.

Barrier	Explanation	Examples
Executive function (memory, planning, organization)	People with ADHD find it harder to plan, organize and follow through on routine tasks	Forgetting meals, running out of ingredients, finding recipes overwhelming, relying on eating out
Hunger and fullness cues	Difficulty tuning into the body's signals	Forgetting to eat until ravenous, overeating past fullness without realizing
Sleep disruption	Poor sleep in ADHD is linked to circadian rhythm disruption, co-existing mental health issues and irregular routines	Cravings for foods, lack of motivation to cook, energy and mood swings
Motivation and reward systems	Dopamine differences can mean food feels extra rewarding especially when emotions are high or when you're understimulated. Low-stimulation, repetitive tasks are harder to start	Eating for comfort, eating quickly without thought. Avoiding mundane tasks such as emptying the dishwasher can get in the way of starting cooking
Activity	Restlessness and high activity mean energy needs are greater	Running out of energy, irritability, concentration dips, meals and snacks don't meet needs
Medications	Stimulants can suppress appetite then hunger rebounds. Other side effects include dry mouth and digestive discomfort	Skipping meals, minimal intake during the day, over-eating in the evening when meds have worn off. Cutting out food groups
Sensory differences	Sensory sensitivities to textures, smells or tastes are common in ADHD	Limited range of food options, difficulty eating out with others

CASE STUDY

Jane's Story

Jane is a full-time parent, a job that she approaches with care and commitment. But by the time evening rolls around, the pressure starts to mount. She's juggling dinner prep, while one of her children is negotiating screen-time limits with the skill of a seasoned lawyer and the other has just popped the lid of the glitter for her latest craft project on the kitchen table.

Even on a good day, the kitchen feels like chaos. A straightforward meal ends up using every pan and utensil. One part of dinner gets overcooked while she's rescuing homework from the spilt glitter. Just as she's plating up, she realizes – she's forgotten the vegetables again.

She serves the children their food, feeling burnt out and overstimulated. But to finish things off, she was planning to eat with her husband when he gets back from work and so there is another meal to prepare – exhausted, with little motivation left in the tank.

At first glance, this seems like a familiar story of a parent stretched too thin. But there's another thread running through Jane's experience: ADHD.

In Jane's case, ADHD makes it harder to sequence tasks – so a simple dinner can feel like a stressful juggling act. Switching between cooking, parenting and tidying fragments her focus. Working memory struggles mean she forgets small steps (like steaming the veg) even when the intention is there. And emotional reactivity, often heightened in ADHD, means the mental noise of the evening can feel louder and more draining.

What helps Jane:

For Jane, knowing that her brain wasn't wired for multitasking or mental juggling in this way allowed her to take a different approach.

Some of the small, sustainable changes she made included:

- **Simplifying the number** of evening meals to reduce decision fatigue.
- **Choosing meals** that the whole family could eat, even if this is at different times.
- **Prepping earlier** in the day when her energy is higher.
- **Using visual reminders** (like a sticky note to mark where she was up to on the recipe) before moving off to do a different task.
- Simply **giving herself permission** to rely on prepared vegetables or batch-cooked options when needed.

When we reviewed Jane's struggles and **focused specifically on** the effect that her **ADHD** was having, **it became easier** to find solutions that made cooking less stressful.

Nutrition Principles for ADHD

The way we approach eating may change with ADHD, but the foundations of nutrition stay the same. Each meal ideally includes a mix of protein, carbohydrates, vegetables or fruit and some healthy fats. All the recipes in this book are chosen with these principles in mind, so you don't have to think too hard about whether you are getting it right.

A rough guide is to include **half to a third of a plate of vegetables or fruit** depending on your hunger and energy needs (with fewer vegetables if you struggle to meet your energy needs across the day due to focus differences or low appetite). The rest of the plate can be **divided equally between carbohydrates and protein**.

A useful approach is what is known as the Mediterranean Diet. This is inspired by the dietary patterns of countries such as Greece, Italy and Spain, and has known health benefits, particularly for heart and brain health.

The Mediterranean way of eating is by no means the only example of a world cuisine that places an emphasis on variety, balance and fresh, minimally processed foods but it provides a helpful framework. It features:

- **Vegetables**
- **Wholegrains**
- **Pulses**
- **Oily fish (sardines, salmon, mackerel)**
- **Fruit and herbs**
- **Moderate amounts of dairy, eggs and poultry**
- **More occasional red meat and sweeter foods.**

Protein

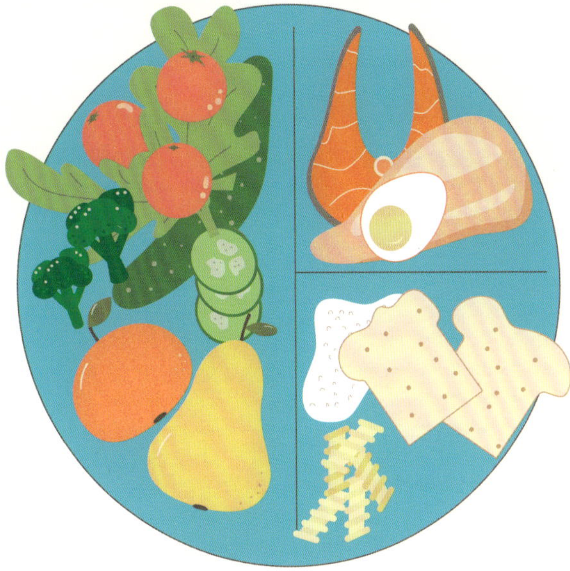

Protein has become a popular marketing hook, but most people actually already eat enough. It's made up of amino acids, which your body uses to build muscle, repair tissues and keep systems like immunity running smoothly.

If you train intensively, are recovering from illness or are an older adult, you may need more protein. However, for most of us, a balanced diet provides plenty without the need for powders or supplements.

Protein-rich foods bring extra benefits too:

- Plant sources **add fibre**.
- Both plant and animal proteins supply **key minerals** like iron, zinc and magnesium which are discussed on page 19.
- Protein also helps you **feel fuller for longer**. It takes time to digest, releasing nutrients steadily and supporting stable energy and mood. This may help you make more considered food choices if you are prone to more impulsive eating associated with ADHD.

For people with ADHD, protein sometimes gets treated as a magic fix. The truth is, it's not a cure, but it may be helpful to include protein at breakfast before taking stimulant medication if you find that medication affects your appetite and makes it difficult to get in all your nutrition through the day.

Alongside fibre and healthy fats, protein steadies focus, appetite and energy, which is why you'll see it woven into many of the recipes in this book.

A useful principle to follow is making sure that every meal and snack includes a source of carbohydrates to keep your energy levels stable throughout the day.

Carbohydrates

While protein is getting good press at the moment, carbohydrates sometimes get an unfair bad reputation.

Carbohydrates are your body's main and most efficient energy source, fuelling your muscles, nervous system and brain. Because your brain doesn't store energy, it depends on a steady supply of carbohydrates throughout the day to **keep your thinking sharp and help your memory, focus, planning and emotional control** – all of which is particularly important in managing ADHD.

If you skip carbohydrates for too long, it can leave you feeling foggy, irritable and unable to concentrate. For someone with ADHD, these effects make it even more challenging to plan, stay organized and regulate emotions.

There are three main types:

- **Sugars** – found naturally in fruit and honey, but also in sweets.
- **Starches** – in foods like bread, pasta, rice, potatoes and cereals.
- **Fibre** – in vegetables, fruit, nuts, seeds and wholegrains.

Fruit and Vegetables

Fruits and vegetables are rich in vitamins, minerals, fibre and antioxidants, all of which help reduce the risk of heart disease, stroke and certain cancers.

Fermented foods like kefir or kimchi can be a nice extra if you enjoy them, but vegetables are far more important for feeding healthy gut bacteria.

The best way to support a healthy microbiome is by eating a wide variety of vegetables and fruit and other plant sources like beans, nuts and wholegrains – these provide the fibre gut bacteria need. Your gut and brain are closely connected. In ADHD, this matters because gut health can affect neurotransmitters like serotonin and dopamine, which in turn regulate mood, focus, energy levels and sleep.

Fats and Oils

Fats are another nutrient group that often gets misunderstood. Many people still think of fat as 'bad', but the truth is that healthy fats are essential for both body and mind.

Fats provide concentrated energy, help the body absorb fat-soluble vitamins (A, D, E and K), and form part of every cell membrane in the body. They are vital for hormone production, brain health and protecting organs. Their importance in brain health has led to extensive research on the role of omega-3s in ADHD, which I will come back to in the section on supplements.

Fats also make food more enjoyable to eat by dissolving aromatic compounds, which helps carry flavour so that it tastes and smells appealing.

There are different types of fats:

- **Monounsaturated fats** – found in olive oil, avocados, nuts and nut butters.
- **Polyunsaturated fats** – including omega-3s from oily fish (like salmon, mackerel and trout) and omega-6s from seeds, walnuts and sunflower oil.
- **Saturated fats** – found in foods like cheese, meat and butter. These can be eaten in moderation but are best balanced with the healthier types above.

Fats are not the enemy. Choosing mostly unsaturated fats from plant oils, nuts, seeds and oily fish supports heart health, brain function and overall wellbeing.

Snacks and Desserts

Snacks between meals help us sustain energy, mood and focus. They are especially helpful for people who find it difficult to meet their energy needs across the day. So, if you are someone who is very active or you have a poor appetite, they're going to be important for you.

It helps to move away from all-or-nothing thinking about food. Labelling foods as 'good' or 'bad' often sets up unrealistic expectations and fuels guilt or shame. Thoughtfully building these into your routine – enjoying them in moderation or placing sweet foods at the end of the meal, where the other nutrients will slow the energy release – can make them feel less forbidden and help prevent unplanned or emotional overeating.

Snack foods and desserts add joy to eating and if meals and snacks never include foods you genuinely enjoy, you're going to be left feeling unsatisfied and more prone to impulsive eating.

CASE STUDY

Matt's Story

Matt is a freelance graphic designer in his early thirties. During our calls, I could see half-finished sketches on his desk, art supplies on his shelves and an array of Post-it notes plastered across the walls. He clearly loves his work, but his days rarely follow a conventional routine.

Nights are often restless. Matt lies in bed scrolling through design inspiration, tweaking sketches in his mind long after he planned to go to sleep. When the alarm goes off, he drags himself out of bed and reaches for his ADHD medication, knowing it will help him focus. Breakfast is quick and healthy – often a boiled egg with toast – and he told me he carefully avoids sugar. He really wants to eat well and start the day on the right note.

Once he settles at his desk, Matt slips into hyperfocus with his design work. Hours pass, and hunger, thirst, even the call of nature, often go unnoticed. Lunch disappears entirely, lost in the flow of his projects.

By mid-afternoon, the first real pangs of hunger hit. Energy dips, concentration falters, and the sugar-free intentions he set out with start to waver. He might grab a protein bar, some nuts, or a piece of fruit – but these snacks rarely feel satisfying. By the time he gets home, the medication has worn off and hunger strikes all at once: urgent, loud and impossible to ignore.

Matt automatically reaches for sweets and quick comfort foods – a chocolate bar, a slice of cake or leftover pizza. Afterwards, he feels frustrated that he couldn't stick to the healthy eating plan he carefully followed in the morning.

What helps Matt:

Initially, we introduced some quick-to-prepare breakfasts and lunches and discussed ways to make eating more automatic during the day. As Matt became better nourished through the afternoon, he started to enjoy cooking more in the evening, playing music while preparing meals and experimenting with recipes. This became his wind-down time.

But over time, he noticed that certain triggers, like someone bringing cake into the office, could still send him on a sugar 'spin.' We realized that the more he denied himself small pleasures, the more intense and uncontrollable the cravings then became.

Gradually, we built in a few sweet or comforting foods throughout the day. For example:

- A piece of dark chocolate with his mid-morning coffee
- A biscuit after lunch
- A dessert with his evening meal

Building these sweet foods into his routine meant that they became part of a balanced approach rather than a 'failure.' This simple shift transformed his relationship with food. Eating is no longer a battleground between discipline and desire; it becomes a daily practice that sustains both his body and his creativity.

It's easy to find bold claims about diets or supplements that 'treat' ADHD. The reality is that the evidence on ADHD and diet is limited and there is no strong evidence to support specific diets or supplements as a way of improving symptoms.

Current NICE guidance is clear: a **balanced diet, regular meals, good nutrition and physical activity** matter most. Eliminating foods, avoiding additives, or relying on supplements has **not** been shown to improve ADHD symptoms in adults.

Eliminations & Supplements

Omega-3 Fish Oils

DHA and EPA are types of omega-3 fats found in oily fish. They are important for brain function and development.

- **DHA** forms the structure of brain cells and supports brain signalling.
- **EPA** plays a role in mood, inflammation and how brain signals are passed on.

They've been widely studied in ADHD – the rationale being that supplementation may help to correct underlying neurochemical and structural differences in ADHD brains. However, a major review in 2023 concluded that the benefits of fish oil supplements on core ADHD symptoms were 'marginal to non-existent.'

Some earlier studies suggested small benefits in young people with very low omega-3 levels, but for most people, eating whole fish is the best option by bringing other valuable nutrients as well. Supplements are convenient, but they're unlikely to make a difference unless you are truly deficient.

Omega-3 sources

Salmon
Mackerel
Sardines
Trout
Chia seeds
Flaxseeds
Pumpkin seeds
Walnuts

Mineral Supplements

Iron, zinc and magnesium have also been studied in ADHD because they play a role in neurotransmitter production and brain function, and some studies suggest they are deficient in children with ADHD.

The challenge is that we don't know if low levels of these minerals cause ADHD symptoms or if ADHD behaviours (like irregular eating) lead to lower intake. On balance, research shows that supplements don't reliably improve symptoms.

The reassuring news is that these minerals are naturally present in many everyday foods. Focusing on variety in your meals usually provides enough. Requirements vary depending on your age and sex.

If your diet is very restricted, checking with a healthcare professional may be helpful. Your GP can arrange a blood test to assess your mineral levels and check for any deficiencies.

Iron	Magnesium	Zinc
Red meat Shellfish and oily fish (mussels, sardines, clams) Legumes (beans, lentils, chickpeas) Dark leafy greens (spinach, kale, broccoli) Nuts, seeds and dried fruit (pumpkin seeds, almonds, dried apricots)	Seeds and nuts (pumpkin seeds, almonds, cashew nuts, flaxseeds, chia seeds) Beans and grains (black beans, edamame, quinoa, oats) Leafy greens (spinach, chard) Avocado, bananas, dark chocolate	Oysters and shellfish Red meat and poultry Nuts and seeds (cashew nuts, pumpkin seeds) Beans (chickpeas, baked beans) Dairy (cheese, milk)

If you've been taking supplements, you're unlikely to have done any harm. But by including a balance of simple, everyday foods, you're likely already covering your needs without the need for expensive extras. The recipes in this book are designed with this in mind, giving you easy ways to get these minerals without overthinking it.

Elimination Diets

Strict elimination diets, whether cutting out sugar, additives or whole food groups, **haven't been shown to help ADHD**. More importantly, they can backfire.

ADHD is linked to higher rates of disordered eating, including both restrictive and impulsive patterns. Rules that feel rigid or punishing often increase stress, reduce food variety and make it harder to meet nutritional needs.

Instead, this book takes a **balanced and flexible approach**. By offering practical recipes with plenty of choice and no forbidden foods, it supports both nourishment and enjoyment – a far more sustainable way to care for both your health and ADHD.

If you do notice that specific foods make a really big difference to your symptoms, it's worth following guidelines and seeking personalized advice from a dietitian about this.

CASE STUDY

Ruby's Story

Ruby is a first-year psychology student, settling into life in university halls. She's joined the uni football club, enjoys her lectures and loves spontaneous nights out with friends. From the outside, she looks like she's thriving – but food has become a quiet struggle.

At home, meals just happened. Her mum would call her down for breakfast, the cupboards were always stocked with snacks and dinner appeared at 6.30pm sharp. Now, without that scaffolding, she often runs on coffee and the odd cereal bar until evening.

By then, hunger hits like a tidal wave. Faced with half-empty packets and wilted veg in her kitchen, Ruby grabs whatever's easiest – toast, noodles, crisps. Bland foods don't appeal though and sometimes she loses interest part way through the meal.

The food gaps soon caught up with her. She had a run of colds she couldn't shake, felt constantly tired and sometimes light-headed. Her parents worried, but it was only at her ADHD medication review, when her doctor pointed out that she had lost weight, that Ruby realized this wasn't just typical student life.

On the surface, it looked like the usual challenge of eating well at uni. But ADHD added another layer: her medication dulled her appetite during the day, her lack of cooking experience made the kitchen feel intimidating, and the demands of new routines made planning and organizing meals far harder than she expected.

What helps Ruby:

With some support, and trial and error, Ruby settled on the following changes that made eating easier:

- Curating a small set of easy, repeatable meals based on storecupboard ingredients that were always available.
- Practising family favourites with her mum during the holidays so she had a few reliable meals.
- Including protein for breakfast, as lunch was her least reliable meal.
- Keeping shopping lists on her phone and popping into the shop on her way home.
- Keeping flavour boosters like pesto and sriracha on hand to keep meals interesting.
- Pairing habits: whenever she refills her water bottle, she grabs a snack for her bag.

Every person with ADHD has their own unique relationship with food, with different preferences, routines and challenges. There are a few challenges that come up regularly with many people I work with, and the recipes in this book are all designed with these in mind.

Six Common Challenges to Eating Well with ADHD

1. Eating Enough Earlier in the Day

For many of my clients with ADHD, mornings and early afternoon pass in a blur of tasks, distractions and demands. Food can slip down the list of priorities until evening, when suddenly hunger comes crashing in all at once.

Medications can make this even trickier, dulling appetite at the very time when the body most needs fuel. Eating little during the day might feel manageable in the moment, but it contributes to fatigue, burnout and often eating in ways that feel less intentional.

Try this:

- **Grab and go basics.** Have a few breakfasts, lunches and snacks ready in advance.
- **Lean into leftovers.** Cook extra dinner so leftovers become tomorrow's lunch or dinner.
- **Back up options.** Stock some ready-made meals or easy choices for the days when cooking feels too difficult.
- **Ditch the boring decisions**. If you find lunch stressful, repeat the same meal Monday to Friday, then switch it up next week. Decision made once, not five times.

2. Planning Meals

Social media and food marketing can make it seem like every meal has to look beautiful, be perfectly balanced and taste amazing. Images of flawless plates and elaborate recipes can set unrealistic expectations, leaving you feeling that quick or simple meals aren't good enough.

For many people with ADHD, trying to reinvent the wheel every night only adds unnecessary decision fatigue. Instead, think of meal planning as building a small 'capsule wardrobe' of meals – a few reliable outfits you can mix and match.

Try this:

- **Create a shortlist.** Make a list of five favourite recipes you *know* you can do.
- **Start simple.** Pick one meal, make it in a batch, and repeat it a few times. Today's dinner can become tomorrow's lunch with no extra effort. Once you've mastered one or two easy meals, then gradually expand your repertoire.
- **Cook a base.** Start with a simple dish and change it up with different additions. A big pot of chilli made on a Sunday can work with rice on a Monday, a jacket potato topping on Tuesday and thrown in a wrap with salad for lunch on Wednesday.
- **Dial the flavour up or down.** Sauces and spices can transform a meal and keep it interesting. Give a simple grilled chicken a new twist with sauces, spices or a side. Sweet chilli sauce makes chicken Thai-inspired, pesto turns it Italian, and add hummus and flatbread and it's Mediterranean. Because sensory experiences vary with ADHD, some people crave big, bold tastes while others find them overwhelming. Keeping a collection of sauces, spices and dressings lets you 'dial up or down' the intensity without reinventing the whole meal.

3. Getting Started

Sometimes it's not the cooking itself that feels like the hurdle, but the small jobs around it. A client once told me that the simple task of unloading the dishwasher was enough to tip her towards a food delivery app.

These small barriers matter – and finding ways to lower them can completely change how manageable cooking feels. Starting a task can be harder when you have many choices or decisions to make.

Try this:

- **Set the stage**. You could try laying out the utensils you need in the morning so dinner feels easier later. It's a little nudge that makes you feel like the cooking is already half done.
- **Gamify clean-up.** If chores feel draining, add some novelty. A three-song playlist to tidy the kitchen or a challenge like 'Can I load the dishwasher before the kettle boils?' might create just enough momentum.
- **Delete your food delivery apps.** You can easily redownload them in a pinch, but deleting them creates a small barrier to ordering a takeaway that might make you more inclined to cook something yourself.

4. Following a Recipe

Cooking isn't just chopping and stirring. You have to remember measurements, hold steps in your mind and keep track of what's next so you don't lose your place or skip steps. When recipes are set out step-by-step in the order you'll do them, cooking feels more straightforward – and this barrier disappears.

Try this:

- **Keep it simple.** Choose recipes with clear, simple steps so they feel manageable from start to finish.
- **Set up first.** Gather all ingredients and equipment before you start, so you don't lose focus hunting for something, or end up in a muddle because you didn't have the right tools to hand.
- **Stay on track.** Use visual or written checklists to help you follow each step and avoid skipping over details.
- **Don't overlook shortcuts.** Pre-chopped vegetables, frozen herbs, pouches of grains, bagged salad or shredded rotisserie chicken aren't 'cheats,' they're tools that remove the fiddly steps. If the choice is between using frozen pre-chopped onions or not cooking at all, the shortcuts win every time.

5. Reducing Kitchen Chaos

Distractions such as a ping from a message on your phone, background TV or even a conversation are part of life and they can easily pull you away from routine tasks. A messy kitchen can make the process of cooking harder than it needs to be.

Try this:

- **One-pot meals.** There are plenty of one-pot meals that use minimal equipment – which means minimal washing up.
- **Keep equipment simple.** None of the recipes in this book require specialist gadgets. Store the essentials (for example, chopping boards, sharp knives, frying pans) somewhere easy to grab, and move the less-used items to higher cupboards or a storage box.
- **Clear work surfaces are key.** ADHD brains can find clutter overwhelming, so give yourself space.
- **Clear as you go.** Before you start, put a big bowl or container on the counter and scrape all peelings, wrappers and scraps into it. That way, the workspace stays clear while you cook and cleaning up is done in one go.

6. Managing Time

One tricky part of ADHD is time-blindness. A recipe that should take 20 minutes can take an hour when you get sidetracked with perfectly slicing the vegetables. The mismatch between thinking a meal will be ready quickly when it actually takes longer can be frustrating and sometimes lead to steps being missed later on or the meal being abandoned.

Try this:

- **Follow the time guides.** Use the preparation and cooking times on the recipes as a guide for how long it should take.
- **Set reminders.** Timers or alarms keep you on track and stop meals from over-cooking.
- **Cook to a soundtrack.** Play a podcast or playlist that matches the cooking time to help keep you focused and pass the time enjoyably.

I've seen so many people get stuck because they feel they have to get everything 'just right' before making a change. What will really make the difference is choosing one or two small things to try and giving them a go.

Not everything needs to be cooked from scratch – in fact, keeping your kitchen stocked with versatile, shelf-stable basics is one of the best strategies for managing meals and snacks when ADHD makes planning feel overwhelming. Having a reliable collection of core ingredients means you can make considered choices at a moment's notice, rather than defaulting to whatever's easiest to grab or whatever craving strikes first. If you're unsure where to start, here are some suggestions.

Some Kitchen Staples

Storecupboard:

- Olive oil
- Stock cubes or ready-made liquid stock
- Dried herbs
- Ready-made pesto
- Sriracha
- Soy sauce
- Curry paste
- Oats
- Microwave rice
- Quick-cook noodles
- Dried pasta
- Dried couscous
- Pouched grains (lentils, quinoa)
- Canned chickpeas and beans
- Canned tuna, salmon or anchovies
- Eggs
- Canned tomatoes or passata
- Nuts
- Dried fruit
- Canned fruit in juice

TIPS: Use clear containers for storing things like rice, pasta and oats so you can easily see how much you have left.

Group similar items together to reduce the mental work of searching for things. For example, carbohydrates such as pasta, rice and noodles; proteins such as canned fish, beans or chickpeas; sauces; spices.

Refrigerator:

- Flavour boosters such as sweet chilli sauce, mayonnaise, mustard
- Bottled lemon juice
- Stir-fry vegetable mix
- Bagged salad
- Jarred chopped garlic
- Jarred chopped ginger
- Jarred chopped red chillies
- Pre-cooked deli meats and fish
- Milk, cheese, yogurt and spreads or their non-dairy alternatives
- Fresh produce for recipes

TIPS: Keep things with a shorter shelf life, such as fresh fruit and vegetables, at the front of your refrigerator so that you don't forget about them.

When you open a jar of sauce or bag of salad, use a sticky/Post-it note or marker pen to write the date that you opened it so that you remember to use it before it goes off.

Try grouping your fresh produce by meal rather than by type, to reduce the risk of items being used before you make the meal.

Freezer:

Your freezer can be your best friend if you keep it organized.

- Frozen fruit such as mixed berries
- Frozen vegetables such as spinach, broccoli, edamame beans, peas, sweetcorn
- Frozen pre-chopped onions and garlic
- Chillies, pre-chopped herbs
- Sliced bread, tortillas and pittas
- Frozen fish (prawns, cod fillets, salmon fillets, fishcakes)
- Frozen minced meat (beef, lamb, pork, chicken, turkey)
- Leftovers portioned into individual meals

TIP: Group similar items together, such as frozen fruit and vegetables in the same drawer, frozen fish in another drawer and frozen meat in a third. Label them if possible.

Here are a few easy meal formulas that you can put together using some of your kitchen staples. These don't require a recipe; you can just grab a few simple ingredients and put them together for a low-effort meal. You can adapt these as you like, swapping out ingredients based on your preferences.

Simple Meal Formulas

Breakfasts

Egg & Veg Scramble	=	Scrambled eggs	+	frozen spinach or peas	+	a little cheese	+	toasted frozen bread
Berry & Yogurt Cup	=	Frozen berries	+	yogurt	+	dried fruit or nuts		

Snacks

Yogurt with canned or frozen fruit

Cheese on toast – Add mustard or pickle for flavour.

Nuts & dried fruit mix

Canned chickpeas, roasted – Drain, toss with olive oil, dried herbs and a pinch of salt and roast for 5–10 minutes on a high heat, until crispy.

Crackers with white bean topping – Mashed cannellini or butter beans with a dash of lemon juice and garlic paste/sriracha + crackers

Meals

Tuna & Bean Salad	=	Can of tuna	+	drained canned chickpeas or beans	+	squeeze of lemon juice	+	bagged salad	+	pitta
Grain Bowl	=	Pouch of grains	+	deli meat/fish/ feta/halloumi	+	veg/salad				
Pesto Pasta	=	Deli chicken	+	pasta	+	frozen peas	+	pesto	+	a handful of cheese
Prawn Noodle Bowl	=	Frozen prawns	+	noodles	+	frozen edamame	+	chilli/soy sauce		
Egg Fried Rice	=	Microwave rice	+	frozen vegetables	+	soy sauce	+	whisked egg cooked through at the end		
Simple Fish Curry	=	Frozen fish fillets cooked with a few spoonfuls of curry paste	+	canned tomatoes and frozen spinach	+	serve with microwave rice				

A Note on the Recipes

To make these recipes easier to follow, we've written them with a few things in mind.

Ingredients

Ingredients lists are written out as full ingredients, **in the order of preparation**. You won't find 'chopped carrots', for example. If you need to chop a vegetable, this will be made clear in the recipe itself.

Any serving suggestions will be included in the tip at the beginning of the recipe or in the ingredients list, so there won't be any surprises at the end of the recipe.

Equipment

Every recipe comes with a kit list so that you **know what you need before you begin**. These lists include the equipment that you'll use for cooking the meal, not for serving.

These are also items that you'll likely need to collect from cupboards or drawers and that will require washing up and putting away afterwards. Colanders and blenders are included, for example, but microwaves and toasters aren't. Oven temperatures are given for conventional ovens.

Method

Every recipe method begins with a bit of **housekeeping**: clear your counter and set out your equipment. If you need to preheat your oven or prepare your stock, we'll let you know upfront too.

Timings

While every recipe includes preparation, cooking and total times. You may wish to allow some extra time for recipes that you are trying for the first time.

Make the recipes work for you

Feel free to adapt the recipes to suit you. Don't worry about 'rules' or 'cheating.' If you need to take a shortcut, do it!

- If you hate chopping onions, swap fresh onion for pre-chopped frozen onion.
- If you have no energy to chop fresh herbs, you can usually swap in dried herbs instead (a general rule is to use a third of the quantity of dried herbs as you would fresh herbs).
- If you're not a fan of canned tuna, swap it for canned salmon.
- If you find it easier to measure out all your ingredients before starting a recipe, do it.

And when you find a recipe you love, mark it in the book – fold the corner of the page, pop in a colourful sticky/Post-it note, whatever makes it stand out.

Cook according to your needs and preferences

On pages 38–39, you'll find a Cook by Need contents spread. Here, we have organized the recipes according to the following themes, which may help you identify the recipe that best fits your preference in the moment:

- No-cook
- 30 Minutes or Less
- One-pot
- Batch Cooks

Living with ADHD means food and eating routines can feel more complicated than they do for others, but it doesn't have to be that way. Once you have a better idea of how ADHD affects your daily habits, it becomes easier to design practical strategies that make eating more enjoyable. This book is here to help with that – offering realistic recipes, organization advice and time-saving tips that you can adapt to your own life.

Low Appetite Meal Plan

Regular and nourishing, if you find appetite low in the morning or midday, this plan focuses on a protein-rich breakfast, regular intake and a more satisfying evening meal.

Day	Breakfast	Morning Snack	Lunch
Mon	**Scrambled Eggs on Toast** (page 51)	**Berry, Honey & Yogurt Pot** (page 66)	**Griddled Greek-style Sandwiches** (page 104)
Tue	**Egg Pots with Smoked Salmon** (page 52)	**Creamy Mango Smoothie** (page 94)	**Griddled Greek-style Sandwiches** (page 104)
Wed	Smashed avocado on toast	**Lemon Yogurt Cupcake** (page 198)	**Chicken & Noodle Miso Soup** (page 100) (chicken from Tues)
Thur	**Scrambled Eggs on Toast** (page 51)	**Lemon Yogurt Cupcake** (page 198)	**Spicy Salmon with Couscous** (page 178) (leftovers from Wed)
Fri	**Ricotta & Blueberry Pancakes** (page 44)	**Spicy Nut & Raisin Bites** (page 84)	**Hearty Minestrone** (page 128)* **Cheese & Chive Crisps** (page 88)
Sat	**Ricotta & Blueberry Pancakes** (page 44)	**Spicy Nut & Raisin Bites** (page 84)	**Hearty Minestrone** (page 128)* **Cheese & Chive Crisps** (page 88)
Sun	Nutty granola, peaches & yogurt	Dark chocolate and fresh fruit	**Fig, Raspberry & Prosciutto Salad** (page 106)

Afternoon Snack	Dinner	Reuse Notes & ADHD Tips
Beetroot & Horseradish Hummus (page 72)	**Pasta Puttanesca** (page 170) with salad	
Beetroot & Horseradish Hummus (page 72)	**Roasted Chicken with Butternut Squash** (page 174)	Make double chicken → reuse on Wed lunch
Cream cheese with crackers	**Spicy Salmon with Couscous** (page 178) Dessert: **Lemon Yogurt Cupcake** (page 198)	Leftover dinner → reuse Thur lunch
Roasted Almonds with Paprika (page 86)	**Chicken & Coconut Curry Rice** (page 190)	
Roasted Almonds with Paprika (page 86)	**Tuna, Spinach & Tomato Penne** (page 160)	Make double pancake batter → reuse breakfast Sat Make double soup → reuse lunch Sat *Can swap for ready-made
Butter Bean & Anchovy Pâté (page 76)	**Salmon Tikka Masala** with naan (page 192) Dessert: **Griddled Peaches** (page 212)	Leftover peaches → reuse breakfast Sun
Trail mix	**Pork & Tomato Rice Pot** (page 176)	

Easy Planning Meal Plan

Reuse and rotate – batch cook basics once, then remix into new meals or packed lunches later in the week.

Day	Breakfast	Lunch
Mon	**Tomato & Mozzarella Sourdough Bruschetta** (page 64)	**Sardine Pitta Breads** (page 113)
Tue	**Berry & Coconut Porridge** (page 46)	Chicken wrap, salad and guacamole (chicken from Mon)
Wed	**Summer Berry Granola** (page 42)	**Chicken Caesar Salad** (page 116) (chicken from Mon)
Thur	**Scrambled Eggs on Toast** (page 51)	Chilli burrito (chilli from Wed)
Fri	**Summer Berry Granola** (page 42)	Salmon rice bowl (salmon from Wed)
Sat	**Mushroom Tofu Scramble** (page 58)	Dhal on jacket potato (dhal from Fri)
Sun	**Tomato & Mozzarella Sourdough Bruschetta** (page 64)	Simple pasta with tomato and halloumi

Dinner	Snacks	Reuse Notes & ADHD Tips
Roasted Chicken with Butternut Squash (page 174)	Guacamole with veg	Roast some extra chicken when making dinner → reuse for lunch on Tue/Wed. Store visibly in refrigerator.
Tuna, Spinach & Tomato Penne (page 160) Dessert: **Squidgy Apple Cake** (page 202)	Hummus with veg	
Chilli con Carne (page 184) with rice	**Squidgy Apple Cake** (page 202) (leftovers)	Make double chilli → reuse for Thur burrito Reserve some granola for Friday
Teriyaki Salmon Noodles (page 150)	Yogurt and fruit	Flake leftover salmon → reuse for rice bowl Fri
Masala Dhal with Sweet Potato (page 158)	Trail mix	Make extra dhal → reuse for Sat jacket potato
Chicken, Olive & Cumin Couscous (page 188)	Muffin	Make the couscous once → have the other half Sun
Chicken Olive & Cumin Couscous (Sat leftovers) Dessert: **Instant Raspberry Sorbet** (page 215)	Plain dark chocolate squares	

Cook by Need Contents

Whether you need to get something on the table in under half an hour or you're looking for minimal washing up, pick a recipe according to your needs.

No-Cook

30 Minutes or Less

One-Pot

Batch Cooks

Breakfast

Serves 4 ▪ Preparation time: 10 minutes ▪ Cooking time: 8–9 minutes
Total time: 18–19 minutes

Summer Berry Granola

Ingredients

- spray olive oil, for oiling
- 100 g (3½ oz) mixed nuts
- 200 g (7 oz) porridge oats
- 1 tablespoon maple syrup, plus extra to serve
- 300 ml (½ pint) milk
- 150 g (5 oz) mixed fresh summer berries (such as strawberries, raspberries and blueberries)
- Greek yogurt, to serve

Equipment

- kitchen scales
- measuring spoons
- 1 measuring jug
- 1 baking sheet
- 1 chopping board
- 1 sharp knife
- 1 mixing bowl
- 1 mixing spoon
- timer

TIP: Reserve some of the granola before pouring over the milk. Store in an airtight container for a week and use for a quick breakfast when you're short on time.

1. **Clear** your counter of clutter and **set out** all the equipment you need.
2. **Spray** a baking sheet lightly with spray oil. **Preheat** the oven to **180°C (350°F), Gas Mark 4.**
3. Roughly **chop** the mixed nuts. Put the nuts and oats in a mixing bowl and **stir** in the maple syrup. **Spread** the mixture out on the prepared baking sheet and **bake** in the oven for 5 minutes. **Set a timer** so you don't forget.
4. **Remove** from the oven and **stir** well. Return to the oven and **bake** for a further 3–4 minutes until lightly toasted. **Leave to cool.**
5. **Divide** the granola between 4 serving bowls and **pour** over the milk. Alternatively, you can **store** the granola for future use. **Add** the berries (if using strawberries, hull and halve them before adding to the granola) and **serve** with Greek yogurt and a **drizzle** of maple syrup.

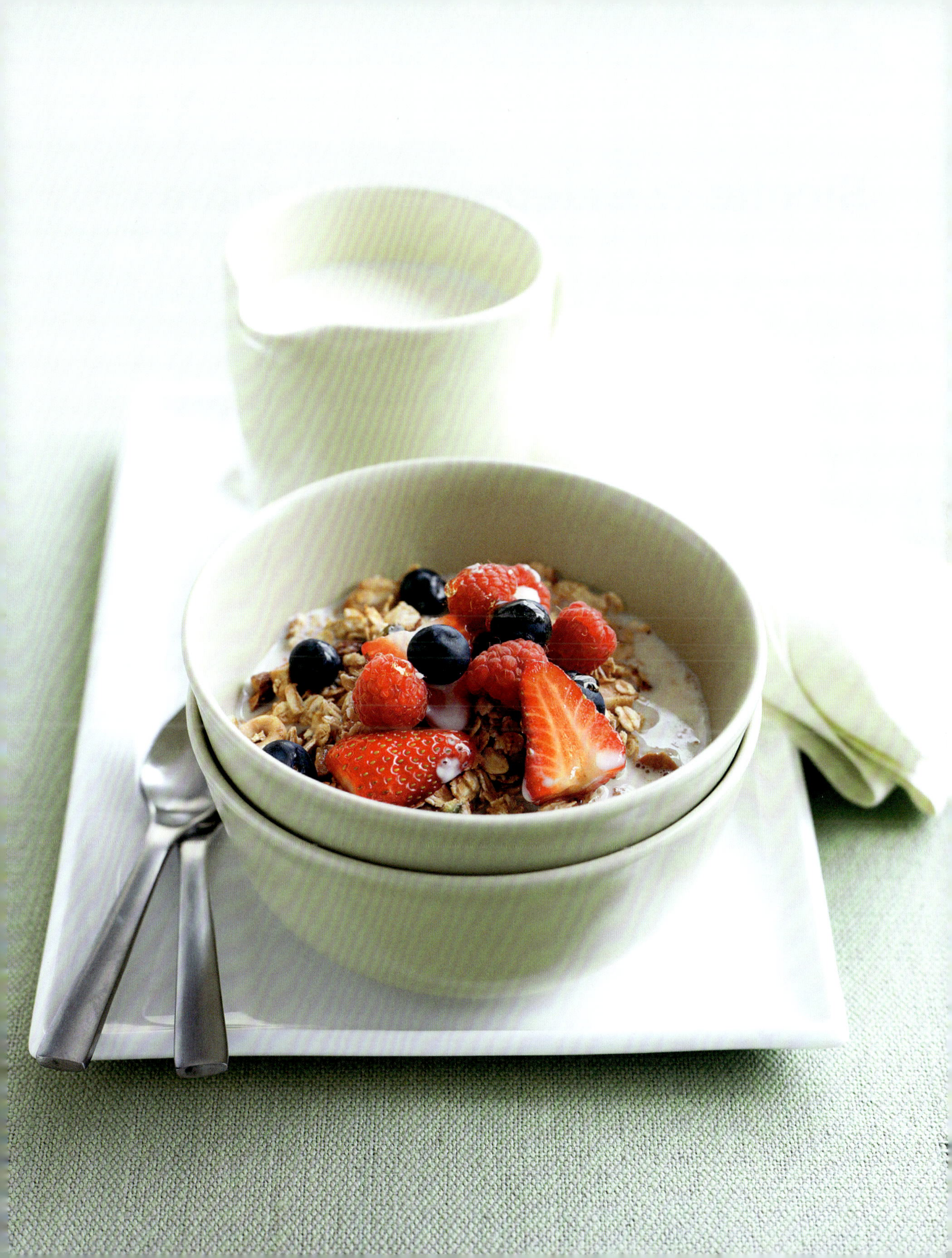

Serves 4 ▪ Preparation time: 20 minutes ▪ Cooking time: 10–15 minutes
Total time: 30–35 minutes

Ricotta & Blueberry Pancakes

Ingredients

- 3 large eggs
- 250 g (8 oz) ricotta cheese
- 125 ml (4 fl oz) milk
- 1 lemon
- 100 g (3½ oz) plain flour
- 3 tablespoons caster sugar
- 1 teaspoon baking powder
- 125 g (4 oz) fresh blueberries
- unsalted butter, for frying
- lemon juice or maple syrup, to serve

Equipment

- kitchen scales
- 1 measuring jug
- 2 small bowls
- 1 fork
- 2 large mixing bowls
- 1 large metal spoon
- 1 grater
- measuring spoons
- 1 hand-held electric whisk
- 1 heavy-based frying pan
- 1 silicone spatula
- 1 baking sheet

1. **Clear** your counter of clutter and **set out** all the equipment you need. **Preheat** the oven to low.
2. **Separate** the egg yolks and whites into 2 separate small bowls. With a fork, **beat** the ricotta with the milk and egg yolks in a large mixing bowl. **Grate** the lemon zest. **Stir** the flour, sugar, baking powder, lemon zest and blueberries into the ricotta mixture until well combined.
3. **Whisk** the egg whites with a hand-held electric whisk in a separate large, grease-free mixing bowl until they form soft peaks, then gently **fold** into the ricotta mixture with a large metal spoon.
4. **Heat** a little butter in a heavy-based frying pan over a **medium heat**. Using about one-quarter of the batter, **make** 3-4 pancakes in the pan, each about 7 cm (3 inches) in diameter, and **cook** for 1–2 minutes on each side until golden and cooked through.
5. **Transfer** the pancakes to a baking sheet and **keep warm** in a low oven while you **repeat** with the remaining batter, adding a little more butter to the pan as necessary.
6. **Serve** 3–4 pancakes per person, with lemon juice or maple syrup.

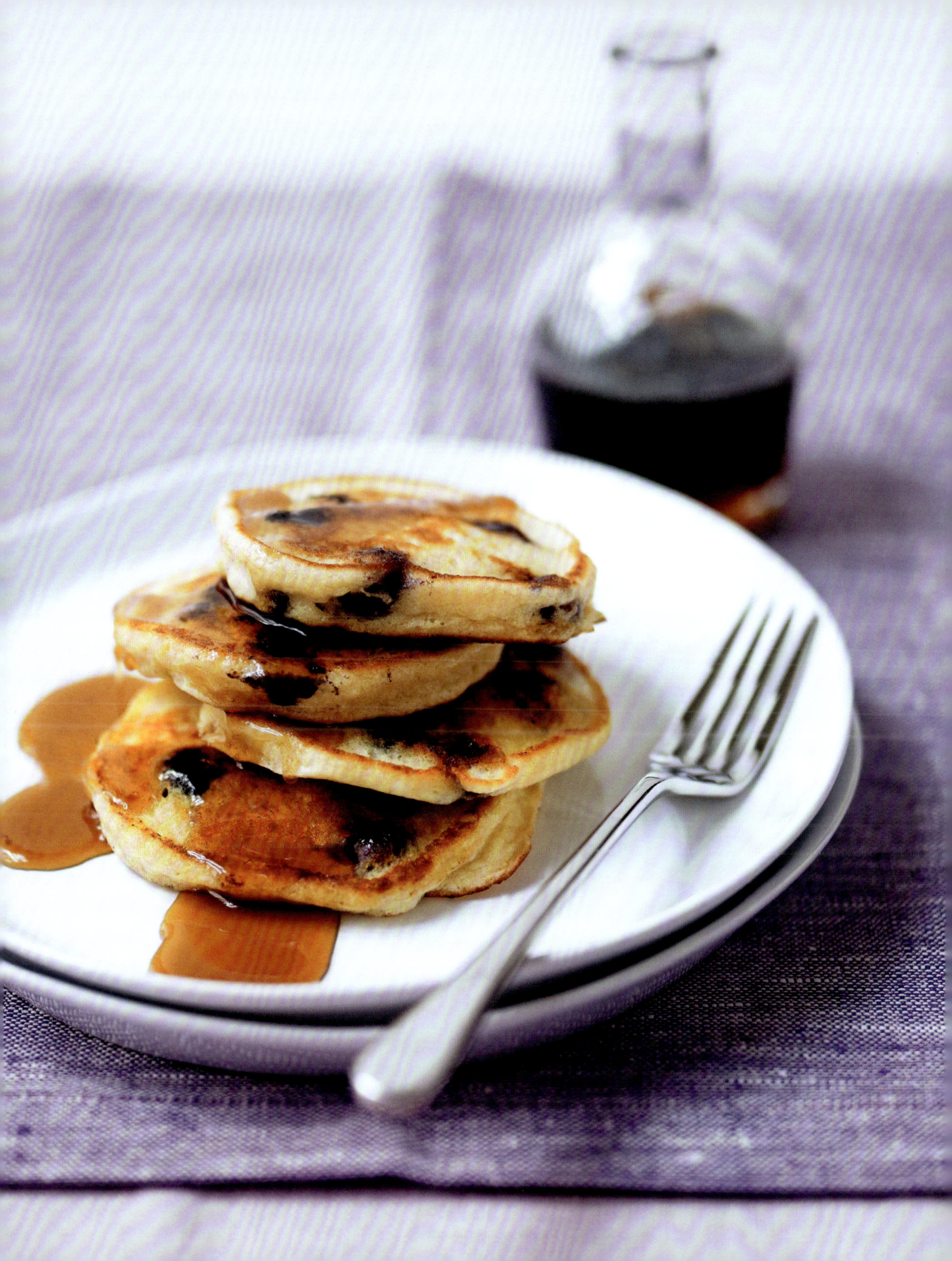

Serves 4 ▪ Preparation time: 5 minutes ▪ Cooking time: 10 minutes
Total time: 15 minutes

Berry & Coconut Porridge

Ingredients

- **200 g (7 oz) mixed fresh berries (such as raspberries, blueberries, strawberries or blackberries)**
- **200 g (7 oz) rolled oats**
- **600 ml (1 pint) milk**
- **600 ml (1 pint) water**
- **4 tablespoons natural yogurt**
- **4 tablespoons clear honey**
- **3 tablespoons desiccated coconut**

Equipment

- **kitchen scales**
- **1 measuring jug**
- **measuring spoons**
- **1 chopping board**
- **1 sharp knife**
- **1 saucepan**
- **1 wooden spoon**

1. **Clear** your counter of clutter and **set out** all the equipment you need.
2. **Hull** the strawberries and **halve** any large ones, if using.
3. **Place** the oats in a saucepan with the milk and measured water. Bring to the **boil** over a **medium heat**, then **simmer** for 8 minutes, until thick and creamy, **stirring** often with a wooden spoon.
4. **Pour** into 4 warmed bowls and **stir** in a swirl of the yogurt.
5. **Top** with the berries and a good drizzle of the honey, then **scatter** with the desiccated coconut and **serve**.

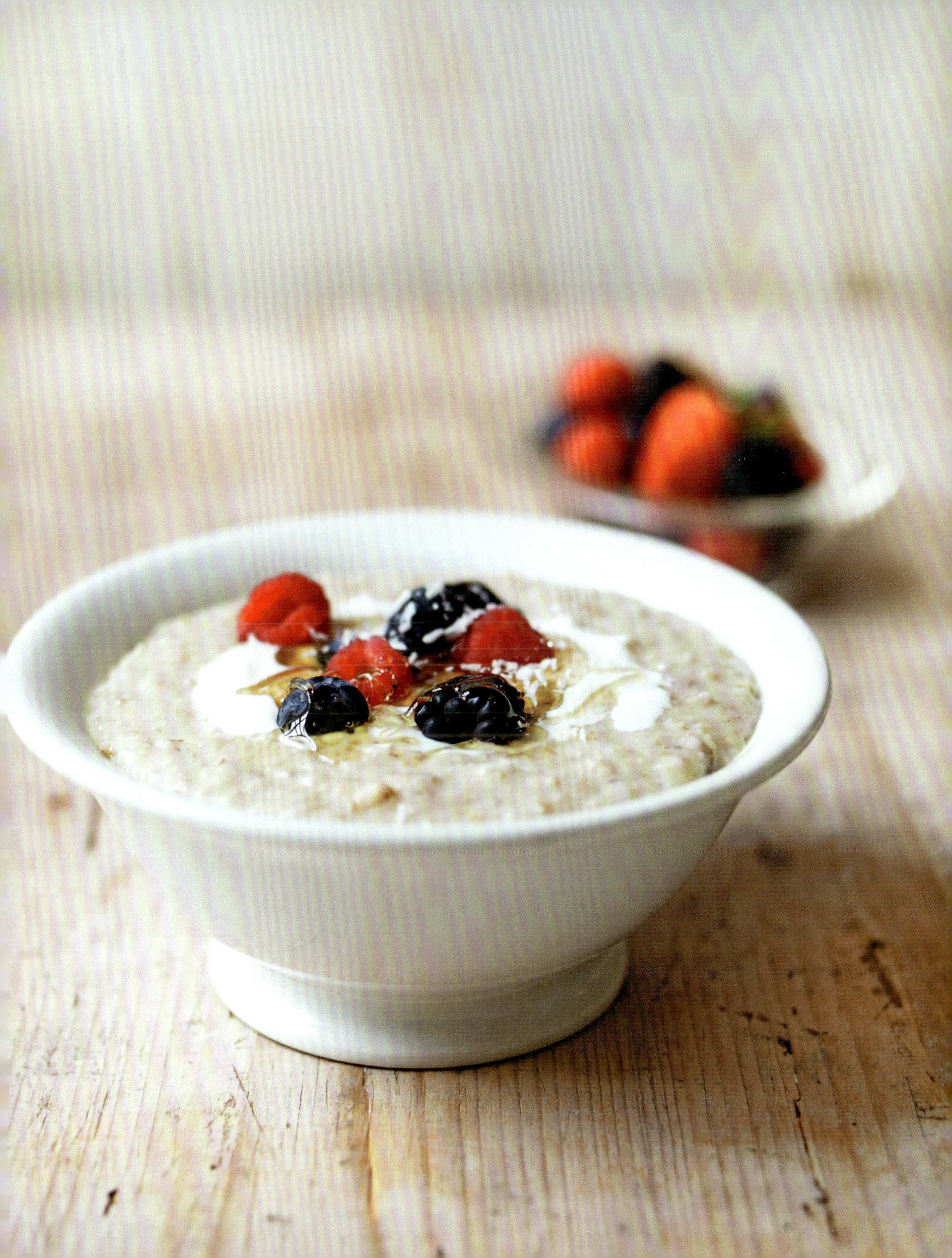

Serves 2 ▪ Preparation time: 10 minutes ▪ Cooking time: 10 minutes
Total time: 20 minutes

Pan-cooked Eggs with Spinach & Leeks

Ingredients

- **1 leek**
- **25 g (1 oz) butter**
- **¼ teaspoon dried chilli flakes**
- **300 g (10 oz) baby spinach**
- **2 eggs**
- **3 tablespoons natural yogurt**
- **pinch of ground paprika**
- **salt and pepper**
- **2 slices of bread, to serve**

Equipment

- **kitchen scales**
- **1 chopping board**
- **1 sharp knife**
- **1 frying pan**
- **1 wooden spoon**
- **measuring spoons**
- **1 spoon**

1. **Clear** your counter of clutter and **set out** all the equipment you need.
2. **Trim** the leek, **wash** under cold running water to remove any dirt and **thinly slice**.
3. **Melt** the butter in a frying pan, **add** the leek and chilli flakes and **cook** over a **medium-high heat** for 4–5 minutes until softened. **Add** the spinach and **season** well with salt and pepper, then **toss** and **cook** for 2 minutes until wilted.
4. **Make 2 wells** in the centre of the vegetables and **break the eggs** into the wells. **Cook** over a **low heat** for 2–3 minutes until the eggs are set.
5. **Lightly toast** the bread.
6. **Spoon** the yogurt on top of the eggs and **sprinkle** with the paprika.
7. **Serve** with the toast.

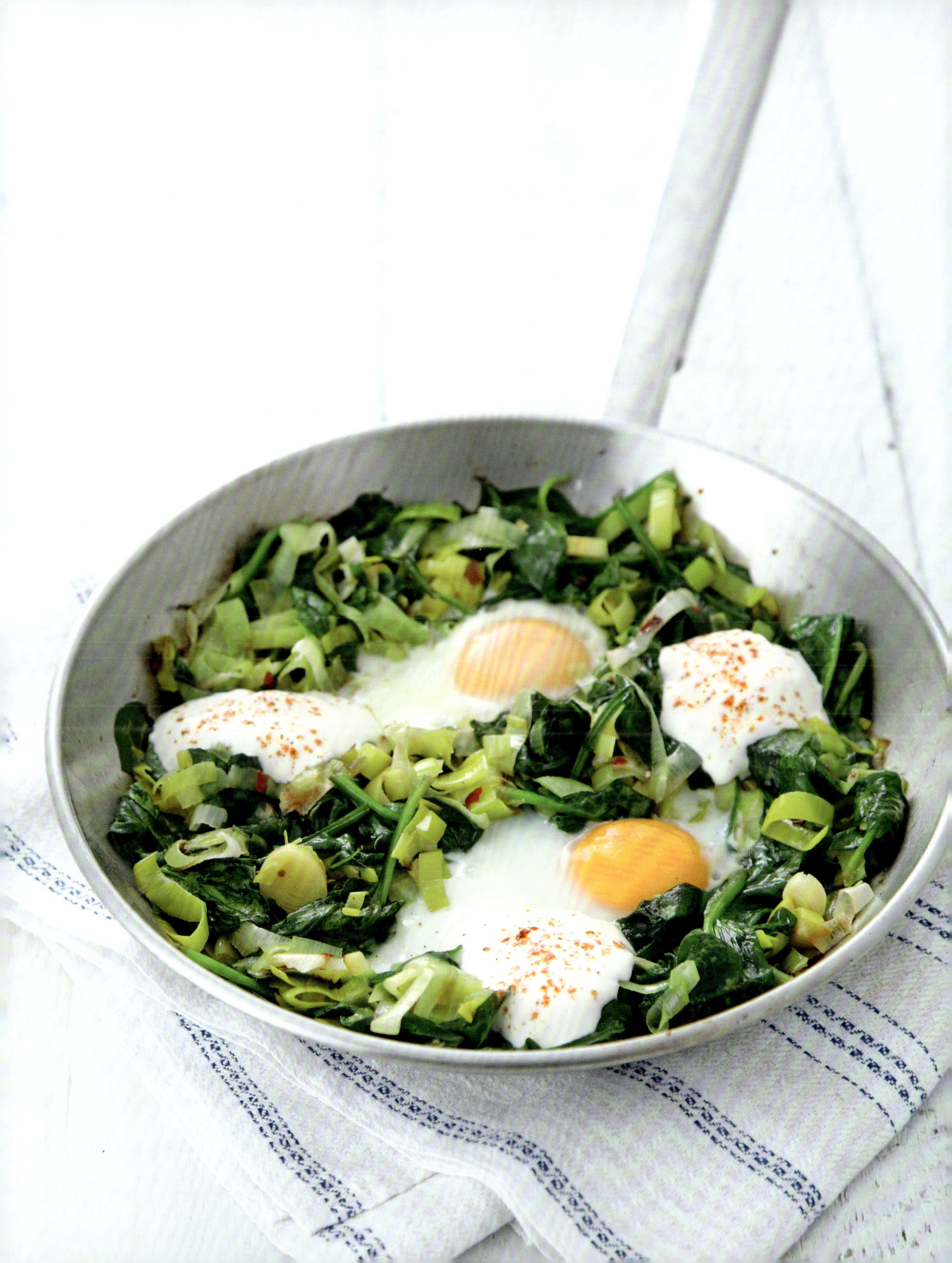

Serves 2 ▪ Preparation time: 5–10 minutes ▪ Cooking time: 5 minutes
Total time: 10–15 minutes

Brie & Semi-dried Tomato Omelette

Ingredients

- **4 large eggs**
- **50 g (2 oz) brie**
- **1 spring onion**
- **15 g (½ oz) butter**
- **25 g (1 oz) semi-dried tomatoes**
- **salt and pepper**

Equipment

- **kitchen scales**
- **1 bowl**
- **1 fork or whisk**
- **1 chopping board**
- **1 sharp knife**
- **1 large frying pan**
- **1 wooden spoon**
- **1 silicone spatula**

1. **Clear** your counter of clutter and **set out** all the equipment you need.
2. **Beat** the eggs in a bowl with a fork. **Season** to taste with salt and pepper.
3. **Slice** the brie and the spring onion.
4. **Melt** the butter in a large frying pan and **add** the egg mixture. **Cook** over a **medium heat**, gently pushing the mixture towards the centre of the pan and tipping the runny mixture to fill the spaces.
5. When the omelette is almost set, after about 5 minutes, **remove** from the heat and **layer** over the brie, semi-dried tomatoes and spring onion. **Fold** the omelette over and **serve** immediately.

Serves 4 ▪ Preparation time: 10 minutes ▪ Cooking time: 10–12 minutes
Total time: 20–22 minutes

Scrambled Eggs on Toast

Ingredients

- **1 small onion**
- **½ green pepper**
- **½ red pepper**
- **½ yellow pepper**
- **1 garlic clove**
- **3 tablespoons olive oil**
- **3 tablespoons water**
- **6 eggs**
- **100 ml (3½ fl oz) single cream**
- **4 thick slices of wholemeal bread, to serve**

Equipment

- **1 measuring jug**
- **1 chopping board**
- **1 sharp knife**
- **1 large, nonstick frying pan with a lid**
- **1 wooden spoon**
- **1 tablespoon**
- **1 fork**

1. **Clear** your counter of clutter and **set out** all the equipment you need.
2. **Finely chop** the onion. **Core**, **deseed** and **roughly chop** all the peppers. **Crush** (using the flat side of the knife) and **finely chop** the garlic.
3. **Heat** the oil in a large, nonstick frying pan and **cook** the onion and peppers over a **medium heat** for about 4–5 minutes until softened. **Add** the garlic and **cook** for a further 1 minute, then **add** the measured water. **Cover** the pan with the lid and **simmer** for 2 minutes.
4. **Beat** together the eggs and cream in a measuring jug with a fork. **Remove** the lid from the pan, **pour** in the egg mixture and **stir** with a wooden spoon over a **low heat** until it is creamy and cooked.
5. **Lightly toast** the bread.
6. **Serve** the scrambled eggs spooned over the warm toast.

Serves 4 ▪ Preparation time: 10 minutes ▪ Cooking time: 10–15 minutes
Total time: 20–25 minutes

Egg Pots with Smoked Salmon

Ingredients

- **butter, for greasing**
- **20 g (¾ oz) fresh chives**
- **200 g (7 oz) smoked salmon trimmings**
- **4 eggs**
- **4 tablespoons double cream**
- **pepper**
- **4 slices of bread, to serve**

Equipment

- **kitchen scales**
- **4 ramekins**
- **1 chopping board**
- **1 sharp knife**
- **1 spoon**
- **1 tablespoon**
- **1 roasting tin**
- **timer**

1. **Clear** your counter of clutter and **set out** all the equipment you need.
2. **Preheat** the oven to **180°C (350°F), Gas Mark 4. Grease** 4 ramekins with the butter.
3. **Finely chop** the chives, **reserving** a small handful to garnish.
4. **Divide** the smoked salmon and chives among the 4 buttered ramekins. **Make a small indentation** in the salmon with the back of a spoon and **break** an egg into the hollow, **sprinkle** with a little pepper and **spoon** 1 tablespoon of the cream over the top of each ramekin.
5. **Put** the ramekins in a roasting tin and **half-fill** the tin with boiling water from the kettle. **Bake** in the oven for 10–15 minutes or until the eggs have just set. **Set a timer** so you don't forget.
6. **Lightly toast** the bread.
7. **Remove** from the oven and **leave to cool** for a few minutes. **Sprinkle** with the reserved chives and **serve** the egg pots with the toasted bread.

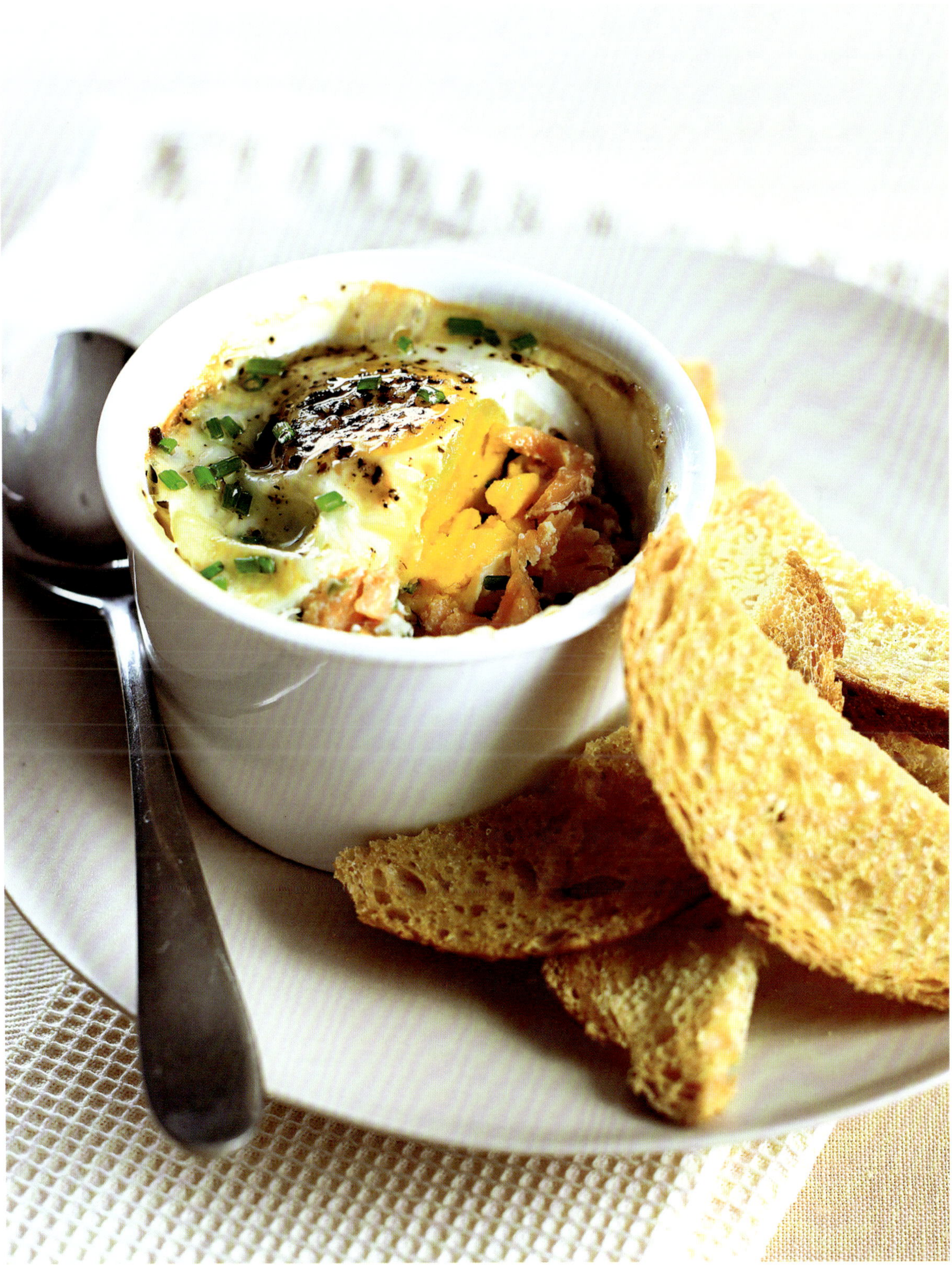

Serves 2 ▪ Preparation time: 5–10 minutes ▪ Cooking time: 10 minutes
Total time: 20–25 minutes

Mixed Vegetable Hash

Ingredients

- 125 g (4 oz) curly kale
- 1 small onion
- 1 tablespoon sunflower oil
- 1 tablespoon wholegrain mustard
- 450 g (14½ oz) shop-bought ready-made mixed vegetable mash, such as potato, carrot and swede
- salt and pepper

Equipment

- kitchen scales
- 1 chopping board
- 1 sharp knife
- 1 large saucepan
- 1 colander
- 1 nonstick frying pan
- 1 wooden spoon
- measuring spoons
- 1 silicone spatula

1. **Clear** your counter of clutter and **set out** all the equipment you need.
2. **Slice** the kale, then **cook** it in a large saucepan of lightly salted boiling water for 3 minutes. **Drain** well using a colander.
3. **Chop** the onion.
4. **Heat** the oil in a nonstick frying pan over a **medium heat** and **cook** the onion for 2 minutes until softened.
5. **Stir** the mustard into the vegetable mash and **add** to the pan. **Add** the drained kale, **season** to taste with salt and pepper and **mix** well.
6. **Cook** over a **medium heat** for 3 minutes on one side until golden, then **flip** the mixture over and **cook** for a further 2 minutes until piping hot. **Serve** immediately.

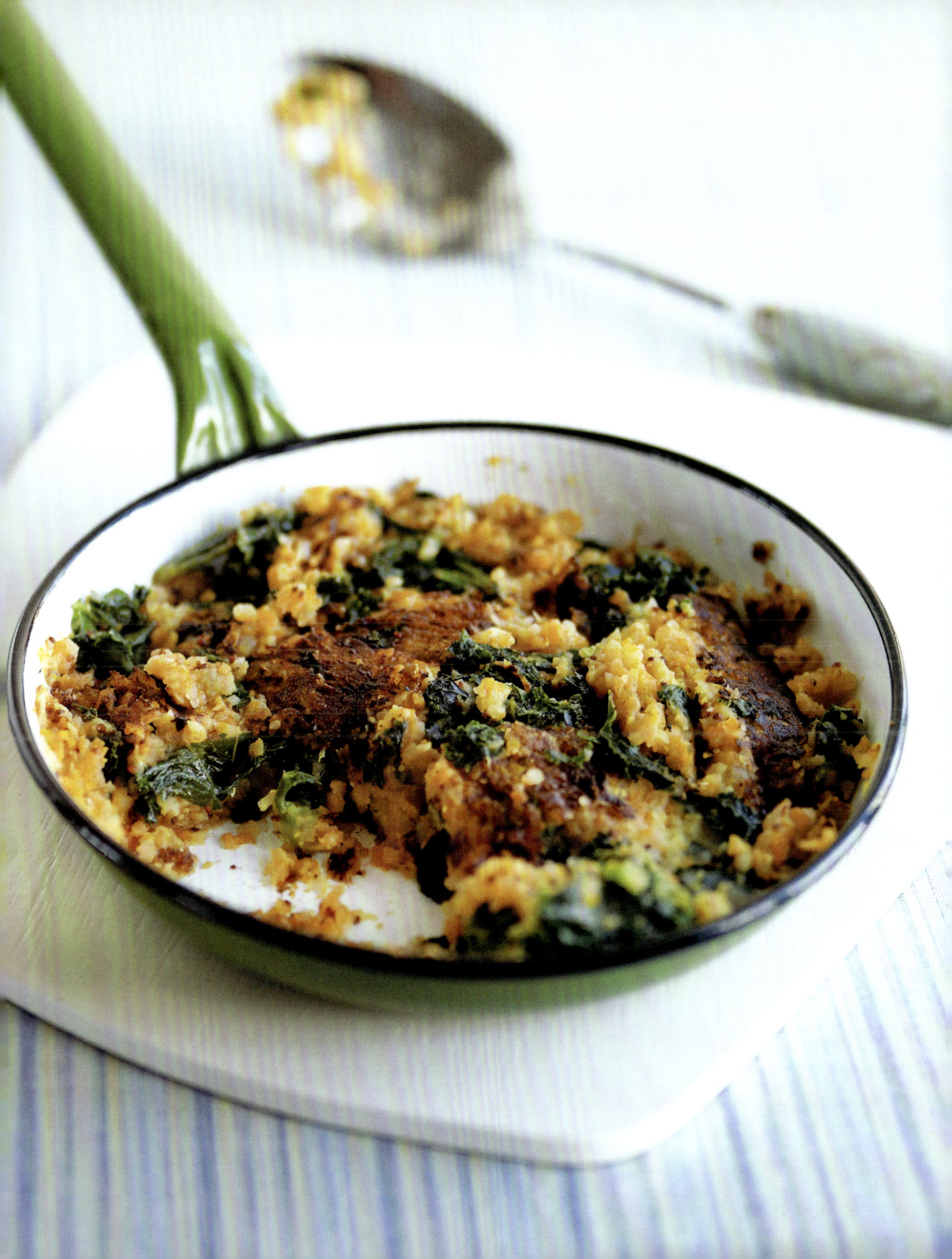

Serves 4 ▪ Preparation time: 15 minutes ▪ Cooking time: 25–30 minutes
Total time: 45–50 minutes

Tomato, Pepper & Egg Tortillas

Ingredients

- **1 small onion**
- **1 garlic clove**
- **1 mild green chilli**
- **1 small green pepper**
- **1 small red pepper**
- **1 tablespoon olive oil**
- **400 g (13 oz) can chopped tomatoes**
- **2 tablespoons tomato ketchup**
- **4 eggs**
- **4 corn tortillas**
- **salt and pepper**
- **smoked paprika, for sprinkling**

Equipment

- **1 chopping board**
- **1 sharp knife**
- **measuring spoons**
- **1 large frying pan with a lid**
- **1 wooden spoon**
- **1 timer**
- **1 spatula**
- **can opener**

1. **Clear** your counter of clutter and **set out** all the equipment you need.
2. **Chop** the onion. **Crush** (using the flat side of the knife) and **finely chop** the garlic clove. **Deseed** and **chop** the chilli. **Core**, **deseed** and **dice** the peppers.
3. **Heat** the oil in a large frying pan with a lid, **add** the onion, garlic, chilli and peppers and **cook** over a **medium heat**, **stirring** frequently, for about 10–15 minutes until the peppers are soft.
4. **Stir** in the tomatoes and ketchup and **season** with salt and pepper. Bring to the **boil**, then **set a timer** for 5 minutes and **simmer** until it has thickened.
5. **Make 4 shallow hollows** in the tomato mixture with the back of a spoon and **break an egg** into each hollow. **Cover** the pan and **cook** over a **low heat** for about 5 minutes until just set.
6. **Warm** the tortillas according to the packet instructions. **Place** a tortilla on each serving plate and **carefully transfer** the egg and tomato mixture on to each tortilla. **Sprinkle** with a little smoked paprika, then **serve** immediately.

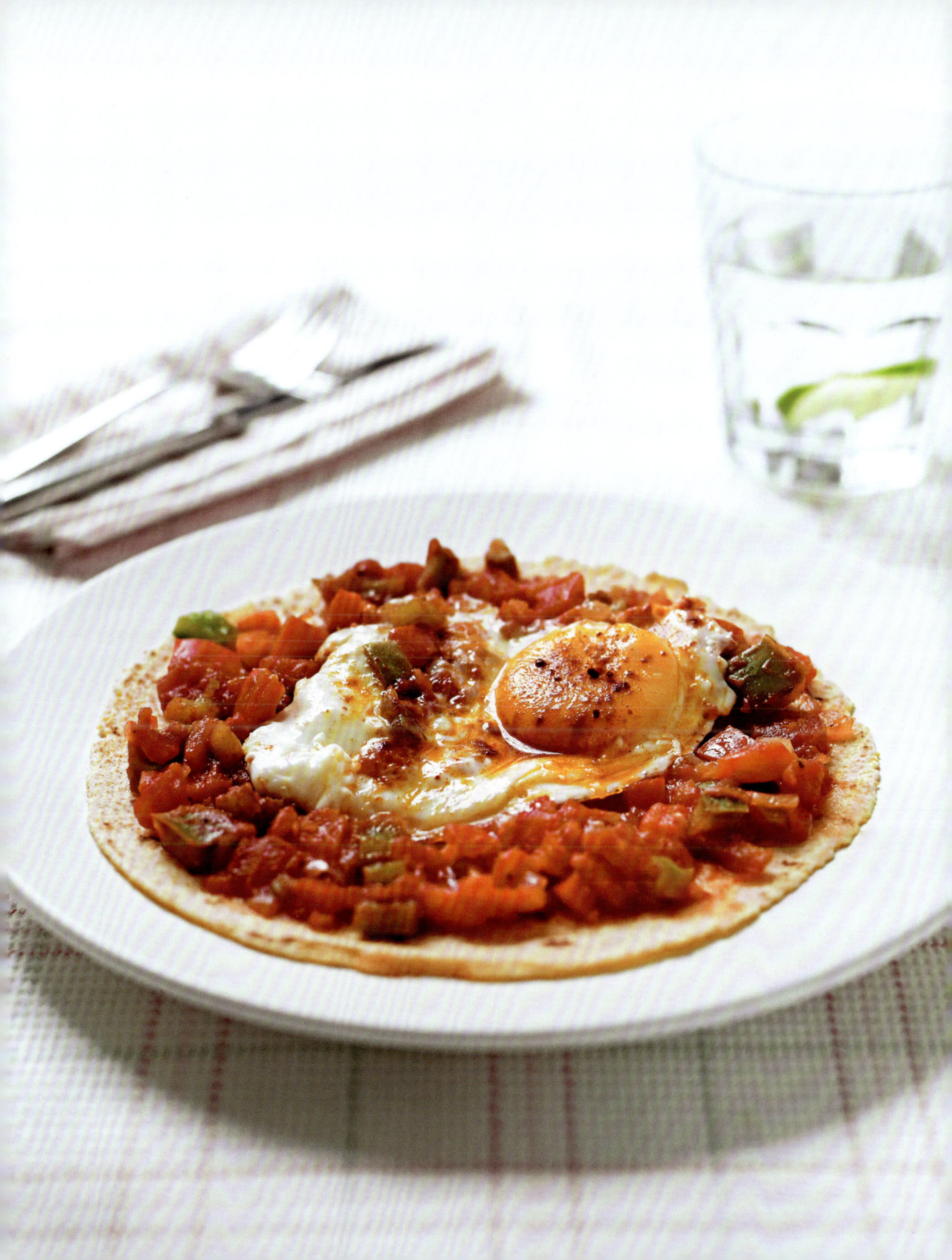

Serves 4 ▪ Preparation time: 15 minutes ▪ Cooking time: 5 minutes
Total time: 20 minutes

Mushroom Tofu Scramble

Ingredients

- **200 g (7 oz) chestnut mushrooms**
- **125 g (4 oz) baby plum tomatoes**
- **30g (1 oz) fresh flat leaf parsley**
- **250 g (8 oz) firm tofu**
- **2 tablespoons rapeseed or olive oil**
- **1 tablespoon tomato ketchup**
- **salt and pepper**

Equipment

- **kitchen scales**
- **1 chopping board**
- **1 sharp knife**
- **measuring spoons**
- **kitchen paper**
- **1 frying pan**
- **1 wooden spoon**

TIP: Serve with toast or hash browns, cooked according to the packet instructions.

1. **Clear** your counter of clutter and **set out** all the equipment you need.
2. **Trim** and **quarter** the chestnut mushrooms. **Halve** the tomatoes. **Chop** the parsley.
3. **Drain** the tofu, **pat dry** with kitchen paper and **crumble** it.
4. **Heat** the oil in a frying pan, **add** the mushrooms and **cook** over a **high heat**, **stirring** frequently with a wooden spoon, for 2 minutes until browned and softened. **Add** the tofu and **cook**, **stirring**, for 1 minute.
5. **Add** the tomatoes to the pan and **cook** for 2 minutes until starting to soften. **Stir** in the ketchup and half the parsley and **season** with salt and pepper.
6. **Serve** immediately with hash browns, **sprinkled** with the remaining parsley.

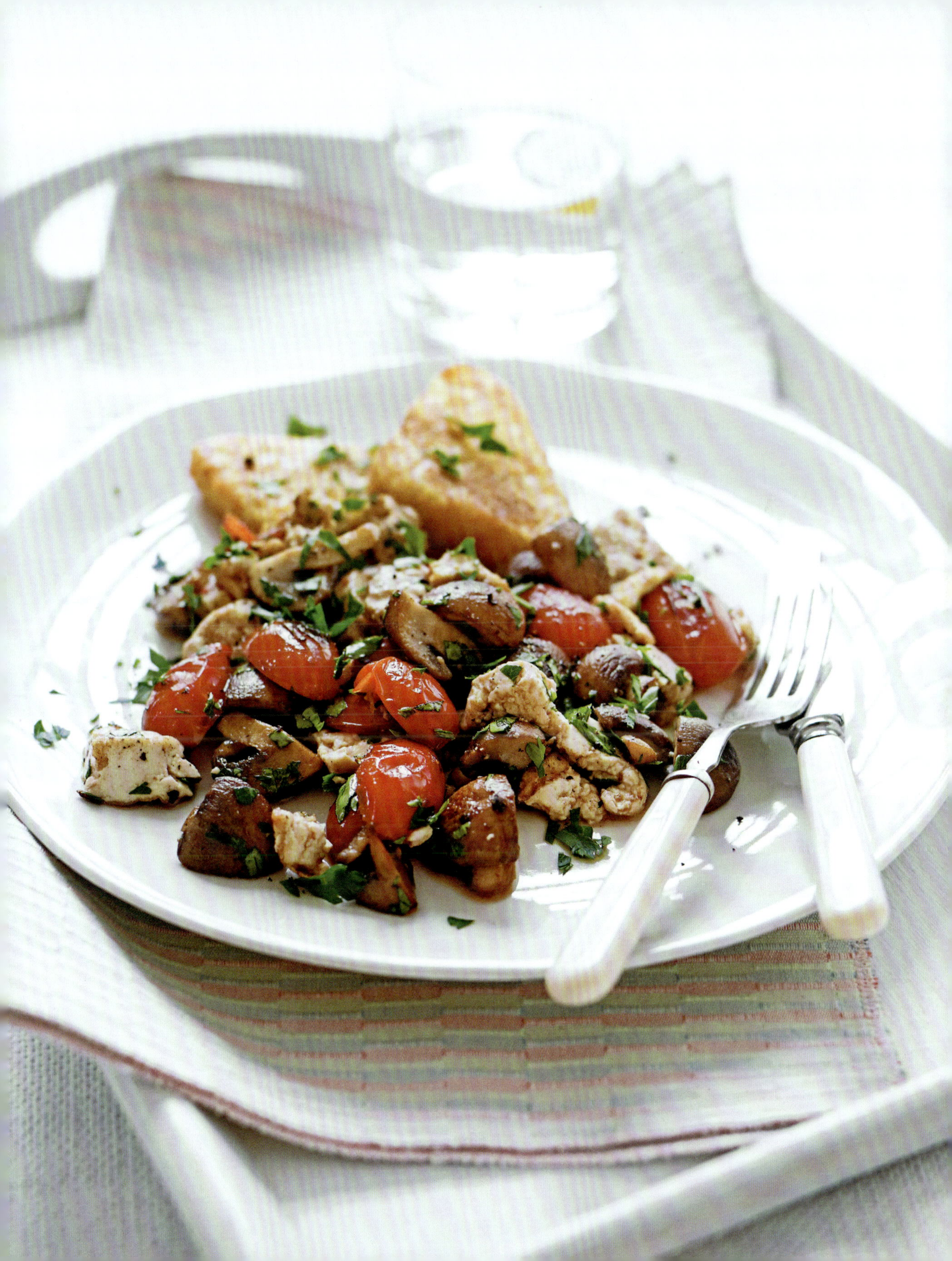

Serves 4 ▪ Preparation time: 15 minutes ▪ Cooking time: 18–20 minutes
Total time: 33–35 minutes

Tomato & Rosemary Muffins

Ingredients

- 3 tablespoons groundnut oil
- 20 g (¾ oz) Parmesan cheese
- 200 g (7 oz) plain wholemeal flour
- 1 teaspoon baking powder
- ¾ teaspoon bicarbonate of soda
- ¼ teaspoon pepper
- 1 teaspoon dried rosemary
- ½ teaspoon onion powder
- ¼ teaspoon garlic powder
- 50 g (2 oz) sun-dried tomatoes
- 2 large eggs
- 275 ml (9 fl oz) natural yogurt
- 2 tablespoons tomato purée

Equipment

- kitchen scales
- measuring jug and spoons
- 1 × 4- or 6-hole giant muffin tin (with holes 9 cm/3½ inches across and 5 cm/2 inches deep)
- 1 grater
- 2 large mixing bowls
- 2 large mixing spoons
- 1 chopping board
- 1 sharp knife
- 1 fork or whisk
- timer
- 1 skewer

1. **Clear** your counter of clutter and **set out** all the equipment you need.
2. **Preheat** the oven to **200°C (400°F), Gas Mark 6**. **Grease** a 4-hole giant muffin tin (or 4 holes of a 6-hole giant muffin tin) with the groundnut oil.
3. **Grate** the Parmesan cheese and **mix** half in a large mixing bowl with the flour, baking powder, bicarbonate of soda, pepper, rosemary and onion and garlic powders.
4. **Chop** the sun-dried tomatoes. **Beat** the eggs in a bowl with a fork. **Mix** half the sun-dried tomatoes with the yogurt, eggs and tomato purée in a jug. **Pour** the wet ingredients into the dry ingredients. **Stir** until just combined.
5. **Divide** the mixture between the holes in the greased muffin tin, then **top** with the remaining sun-dried tomatoes and grated cheese. **Bake** in the oven for 18–20 minutes, or until a skewer inserted into one of the muffins comes out clean.
6. **Leave to cool** for a few minutes, then **serve**.

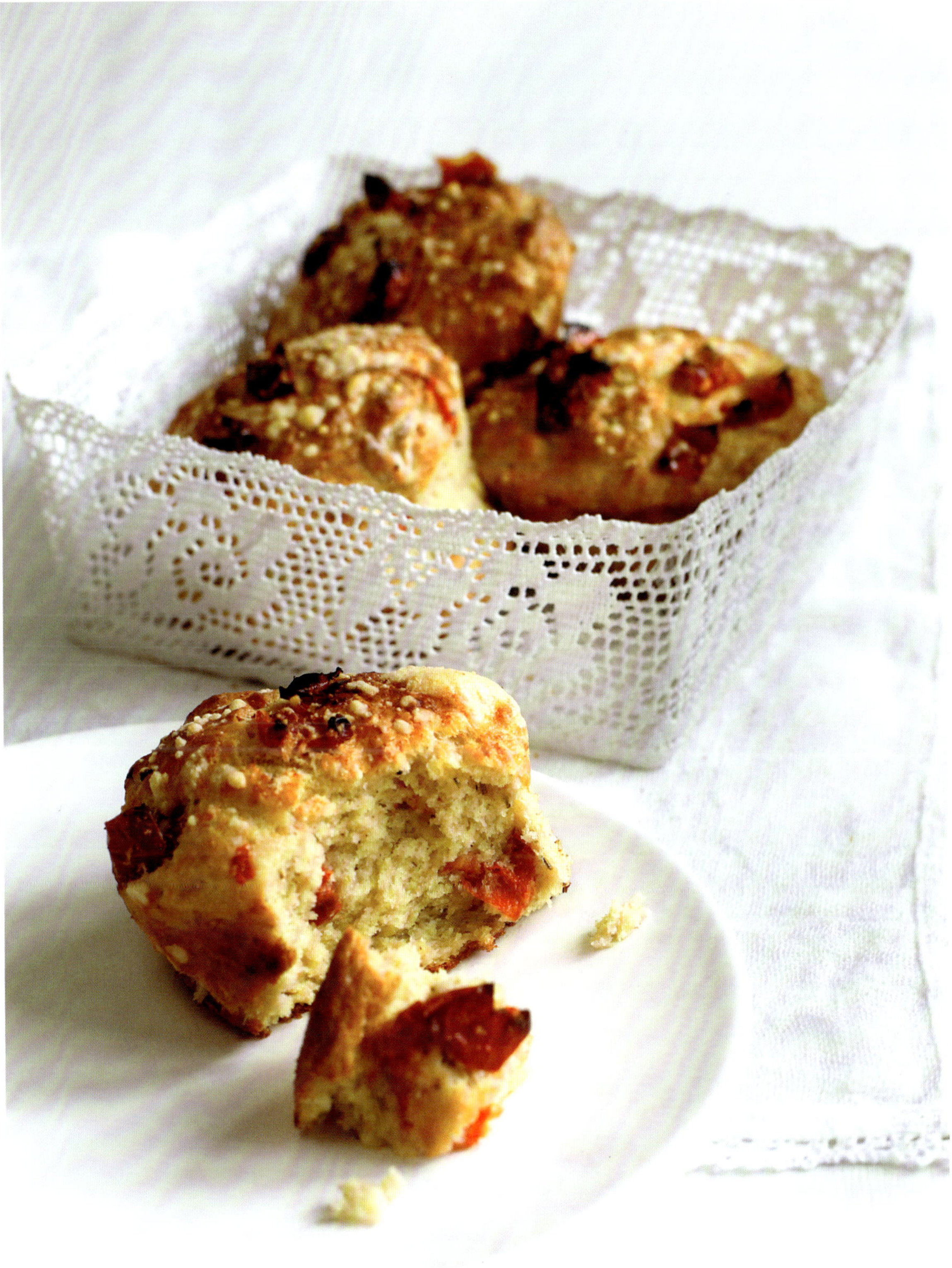

Serves 4 ▪ Preparation time: 10 minutes ▪ Cooking time: 10 minutes
Total time: 20 minutes

Mediterranean Beans

Ingredients

- 1 red onion
- 1 garlic clove
- 75 g (3 oz) cherry tomatoes
- 20 g (¾ oz) fresh sage
- 400 g (13 oz) can cannellini beans
- 2 tablespoons extra virgin olive oil
- ½ teaspoon cumin seeds
- 25 g (1 oz) Manchego cheese
- salt and pepper
- 4 slices of crusty bread, to serve

Equipment

- kitchen scales
- 1 chopping board
- 1 sharp knife
- can opener
- 1 colander
- 1 large frying pan
- measuring spoons
- 1 wooden spoon
- 1 grater

1. **Clear** your counter of clutter and **set out** all the equipment you need.
2. **Dice** the red onion. **Crush** (using the flat side of the knife) and **finely chop** the garlic. **Quarter** the cherry tomatoes. **Chop** the sage.
3. **Drain** and **rinse** the cannellini beans in a colander.
4. **Heat** the oil in a large frying pan, **add** the red onion and **cook** over a **medium heat** for 1–2 minutes. **Add** the garlic and cumin seeds and **cook** for a further 2–3 minutes.
5. **Add** the beans and **mix** well to allow them to soak up the flavours, then **add** the tomatoes. **Stir** in the sage, **season** with salt and pepper and **heat** through, for 5 minutes.
6. **Grate** the cheese and **toast** the bread.
7. **Serve** the toast topped with the beans and a **sprinkling** of the grated cheese.

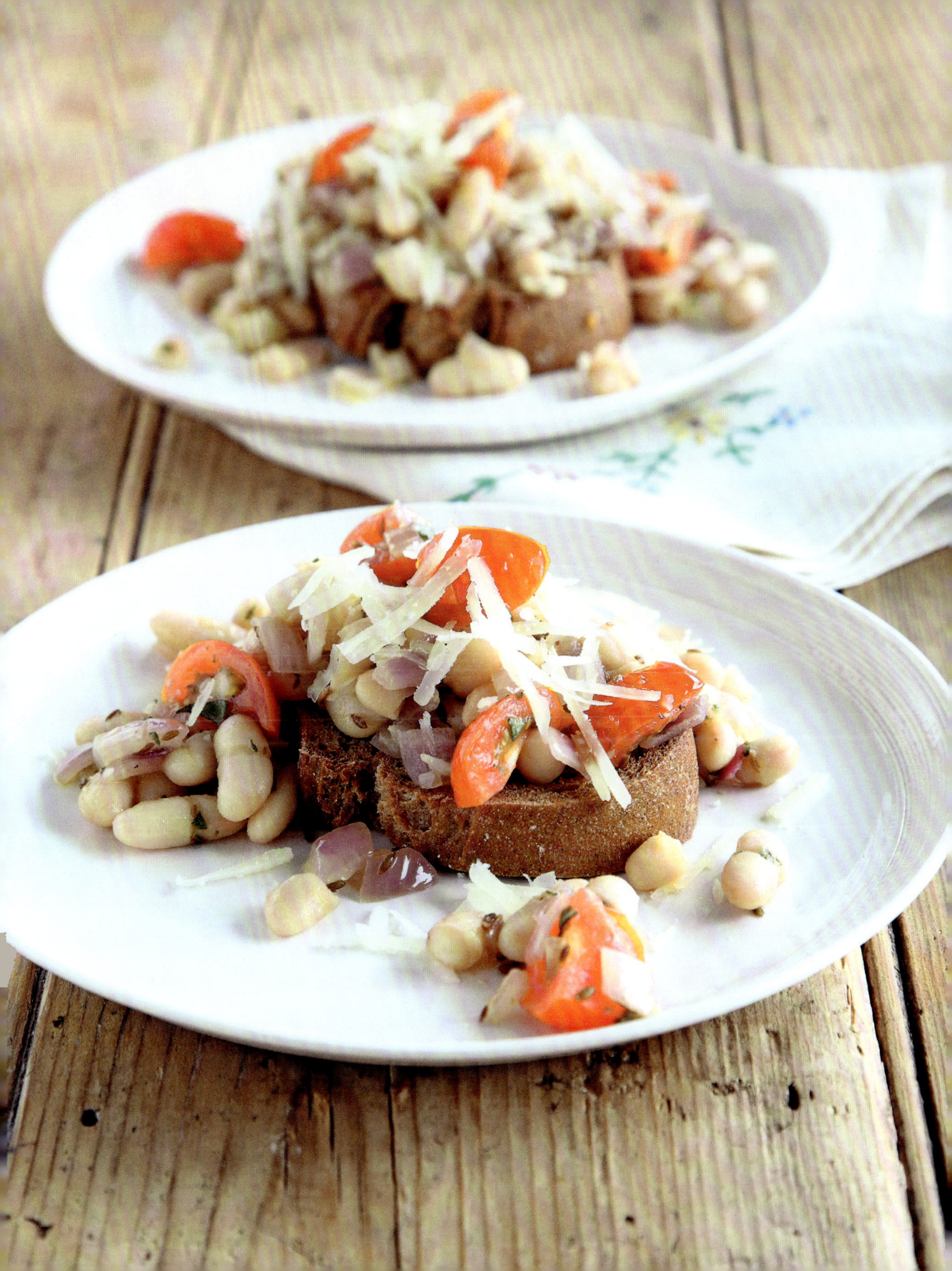

Serves 2 ▪ Preparation time: 10 minutes ▪ Cooking time: 10 minutes
Total time: 20 minutes

Tomato & Mozzarella Sourdough Bruschetta

Ingredients

- 1 small red onion
- 175 g (6 oz) baby plum tomatoes
- 125 g (4 oz) pot mozzarella pearls
- 4 tablespoons olive oil
- ½ teaspoon cumin seeds
- 2 thick slices of sourdough bread
- ½ teaspoon sea salt flakes
- 10 g (¼ oz) fresh coriander leaves, to garnish
- pepper

Equipment

- kitchen scales
- 1 chopping board
- 1 sharp knife
- 1 frying pan
- measuring spoons
- 1 wooden spoon
- 1 pastry brush

1. **Clear** your counter of clutter and **set out** all the equipment you need.
2. **Cut** the red onion into slim wedges. **Halve** the tomatoes.
3. **Drain** the mozzarella pearls.
4. **Heat** 2 tablespoons of the oil in a frying pan, **add** the red onion and cumin seeds and cook over a **medium heat** for 5 minutes, **stirring** occasionally, until golden and softened.
5. **Add** the tomatoes and **cook** for a further 1 minute, taking care not to let them lose their shape. **Add** the mozzarella pearls and **remove** the pan from the heat, **shaking** it a little to warm the cheese very slightly.
6. **Toast** the sourdough slices, then **brush** with the remaining oil and **sprinkle** with the sea salt flakes.
7. **Chop** the coriander leaves.
8. **Divide** the tomato mixture between the toasts, **scatter** with the coriander and a grind of pepper, then **serve**.

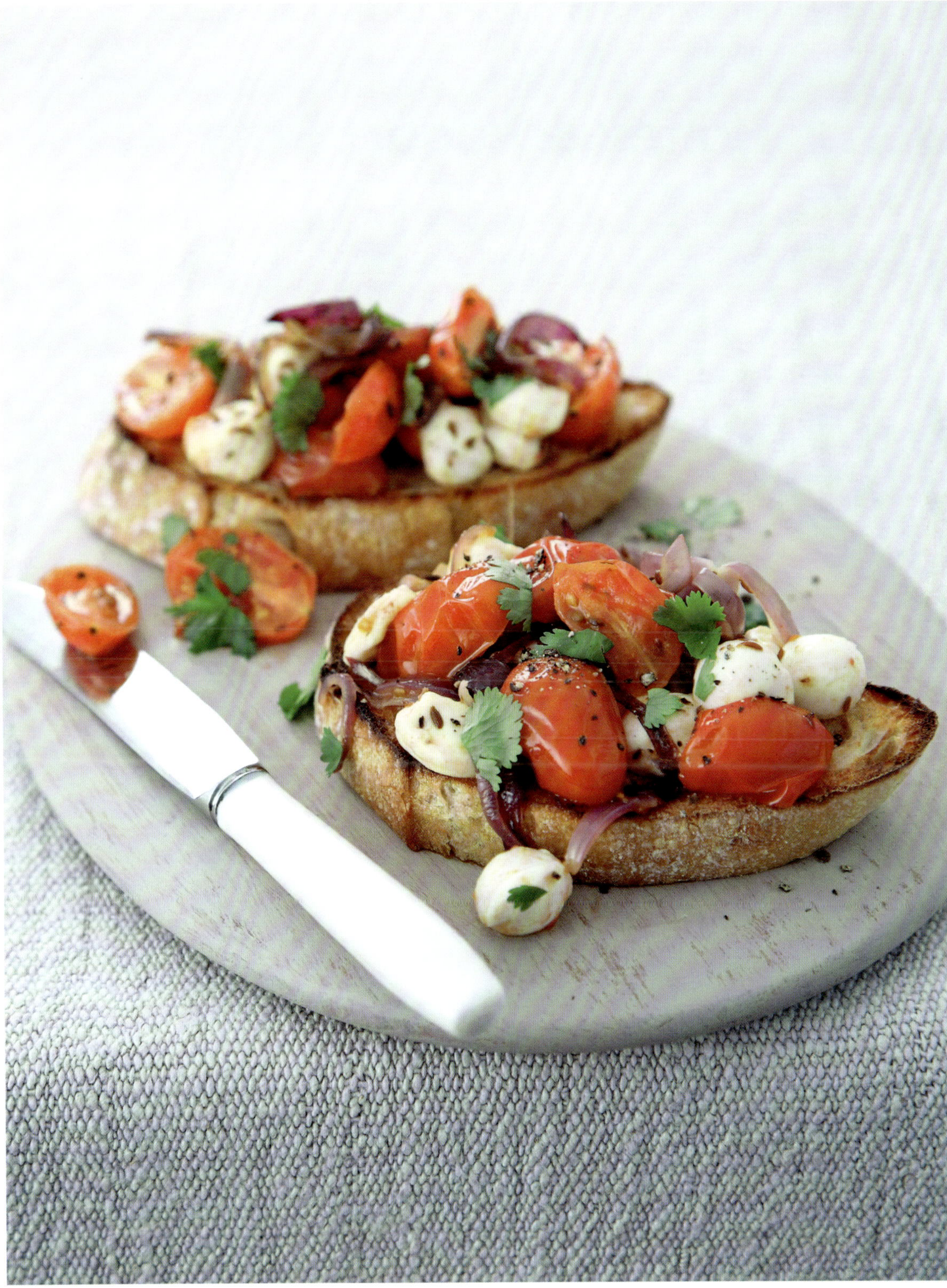

Serves 4 ▪ Preparation time: 10 minutes ▪ Cooking time: None
Total time: 10 minutes

Berry, Honey & Yogurt Pots

Ingredients

- **400 g (13 oz) frozen mixed berries**
- **1 orange**
- **6 tablespoons clear honey**
- **400 ml (14 fl oz) vanilla yogurt**
- **50 g (2 oz) granola**

Equipment

- **kitchen scales**
- **1 measuring jug**
- **1 lemon juicer**
- **measuring spoons**
- **1 blender**
- **1 mixing bowl**
- **1 wooden spoon**
- **2 spoons**

TIP: If you don't have a microwave, defrost your frozen berries in the refrigerator overnight before making this recipe.

1. **Clear** your counter of clutter and **set out** all the equipment you need.
2. **Defrost** the frozen berries in the microwave, on a **medium heat** for 1–2 minutes.
3. **Halve** and **juice** the orange, then **blitz** the juice, berries and honey in a blender until smooth.
4. **Transfer** to a mixing bowl and **stir** in the remaining berries.
5. **Divide** one-third of the berry mixture between 4 dessert glasses or small bowls. With a separate spoon, **top** with half the yogurt.
6. **Layer** with half the remaining berry mixture and **top** with the remaining yogurt.
7. **Top** with the remaining berry mixture and **sprinkle** over the granola just before serving.

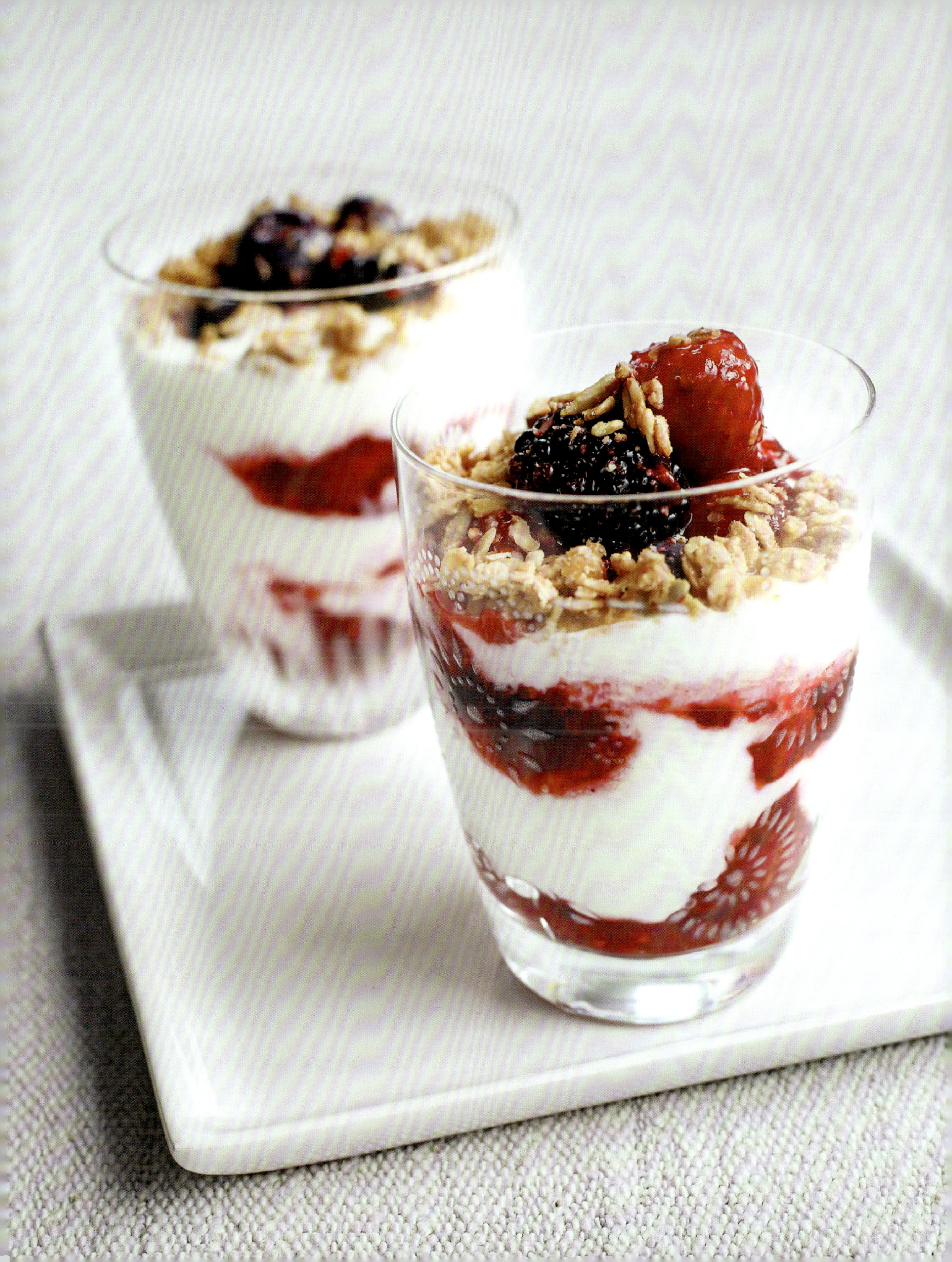

Snacks, Dips & Smoothies

Serves 4 ▪ Preparation time: 15 minutes ▪ Cooking time: None
Total time: 15 minutes

Veggie Snack Plate

Ingredients

- **2 large, firm, ripe avocados**
- **½ small red onion**
- **30 g (1 oz) fresh coriander**
- **1 lime**
- **¼ teaspoon garlic powder**
- **¼ teaspoon celery salt**
- **pinch of cayenne**
- **½ teaspoon paprika**
- **3 tomatoes**
- **few dashes of Tabasco sauce (optional)**
- **2 carrots**
- **4 celery sticks**
- **1 small cauliflower**
- **8 radishes**
- **125 g (4 oz) baby sweetcorn**
- **salt and pepper**

Equipment

- **kitchen scales**
- **1 chopping board**
- **1 sharp knife**
- **1 small mixing bowl**
- **1 fork**
- **1 lemon juicer**
- **measuring spoons**
- **1 mixing spoon**
- **1 vegetable peeler**

TIP: You can save time by buying pre-chopped vegetables such as carrot or cucumber sticks.

1. **Clear** your counter of clutter and **set out** all the equipment you need.
2. **Halve** the avocados and **remove** the stones, then **spoon** out the flesh into a small mixing bowl and **mash** with the back of a fork to break it up.
3. **Finely chop** the red onion and coriander.
4. **Halve** and **juice** the lime, then **add** 2 tablespoons of the juice to the avocado along with the red onion, coriander, garlic powder, celery salt and spices. **Mix** until almost smooth, with some small lumps, then **season** with salt and pepper.
5. **Quarter**, **deseed** and **finely chop** the tomatoes, then **stir** them into the avocado mixture. **Add** the Tabasco sauce, if using.
6. **Peel** the carrots, then **cut** the carrots and celery sticks into batons. **Cut** the cauliflower into florets and **trim** and **halve** the radishes.
7. **Scoop** the avocado dip into a serving bowl and **place** on a platter with the selection of raw vegetables **arranged** alongside.

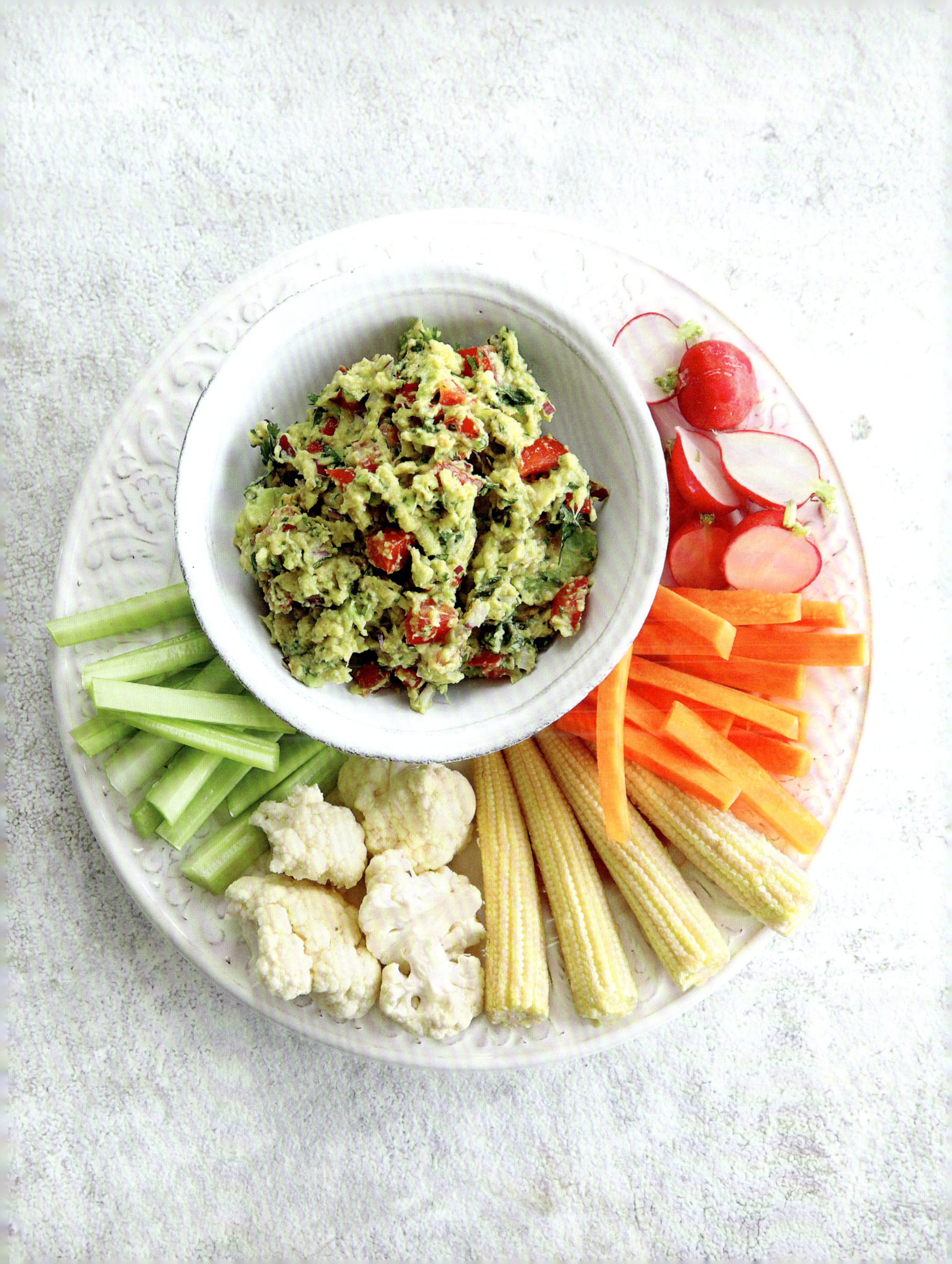

Serves 4–6 ▪ Preparation time: 10 minutes ▪ Cooking time: None
Total time: 10 minutes

Beetroot & Horseradish Hummus

Ingredients

- **300 g (10 oz) cooked beetroot**
- **½ lemon**
- **400 g (13 oz) can chickpeas**
- **2 tablespoons horseradish sauce**
- **½ teaspoon ground cumin**
- **2 tablespoons olive oil**
- **salt and pepper**
- **handful of fresh chives, to garnish**
- **pitta breads, to serve**
- **crème fraîche, to serve (optional)**

Equipment

- **kitchen scales**
- **1 chopping board**
- **1 sharp knife**
- **1 lemon juicer**
- **can opener**
- **1 colander**
- **1 food processor**
- **measuring spoons**
- **1 spoon**

TIP: Store the hummus in an airtight container in the refrigerator for up to 5 days for a quick snack option.

1. **Clear** your counter of clutter and **set out** all the equipment you need.
2. **Roughly dice** the cooked beetroot. **Juice** the lemon.
3. **Drain** and **rinse** the chickpeas in a colander.
4. **Place** all the diced beetroot in a food processor with the horseradish, chickpeas, cumin, olive oil, lemon juice and a generous pinch of salt and pepper. **Blend** until almost smooth.
5. **Chop** the chives. **Cut** the pitta breads into strips.
6. **Spoon** the hummus into a serving bowl and **top** with a dollop of crème fraîche, if desired. **Garnish** with the chopped chives and **serve** with strips of pitta bread.

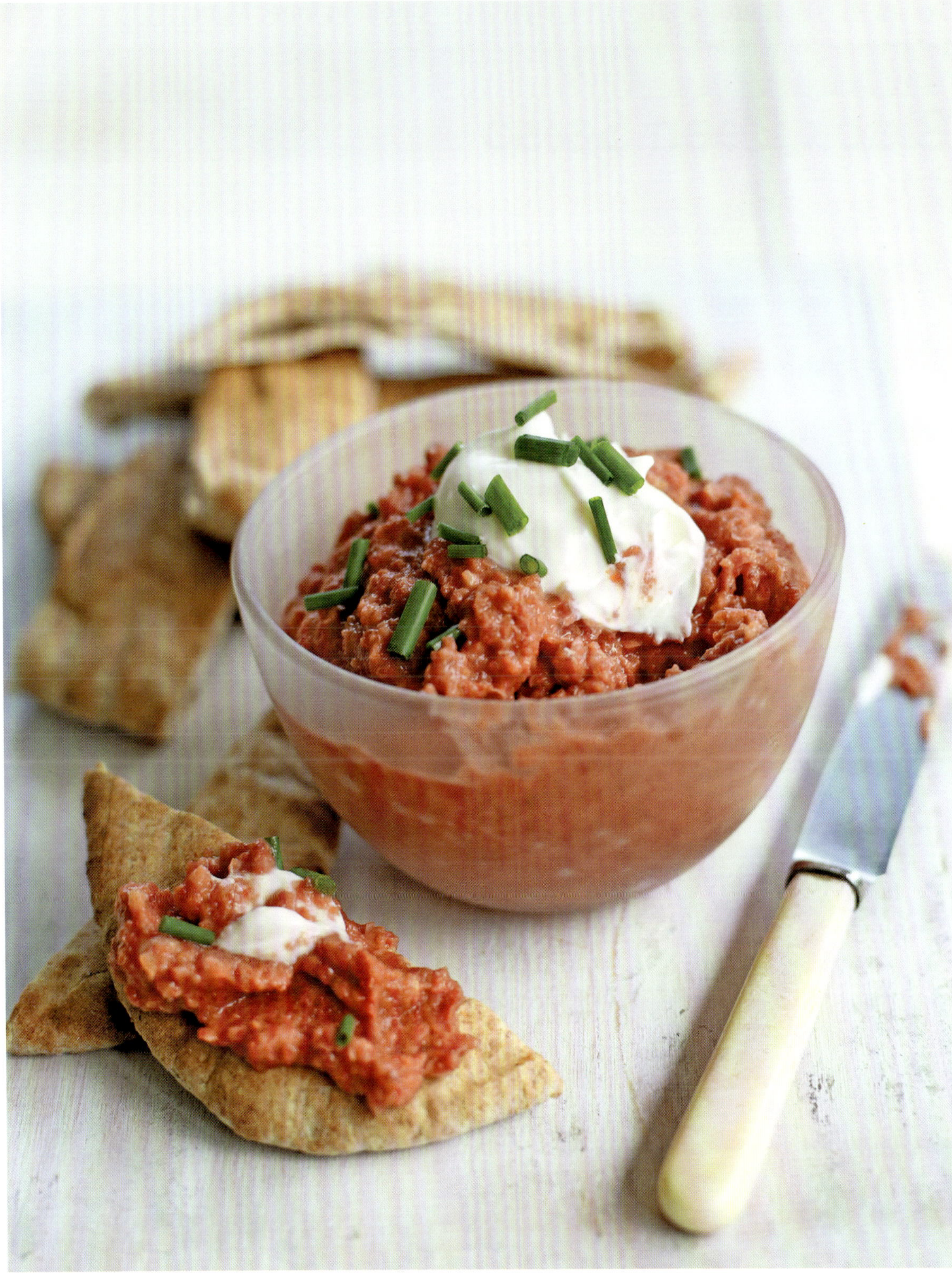

Serves 4 ▪ Preparation time: 10 minutes ▪ Cooking time: None
Total time: 10 minutes

Black Bean Salsa

Ingredients

- 125 g (4 oz) cherry tomatoes
- 2 spring onions
- 1 fresh jalapeño chilli
- handful of fresh coriander leaves
- ½ lime
- 400 g (13 oz) can black beans
- 2 tablespoons olive oil
- salt and pepper
- tortilla chips, to serve

Equipment

- kitchen scales
- 1 chopping board
- 1 sharp knife
- 1 grater
- 1 lemon juicer
- can opener
- 1 colander
- measuring spoons
- 1 bowl
- 1 mixing spoon

1. **Clear** your counter of clutter and **set out** all the equipment you need.
2. **Quarter** the cherry tomatoes and **finely slice** the spring onions. **Finely chop** the chilli, discarding the seeds if you like. **Chop** the coriander. **Grate** the lime rind and **juice** the lime.
3. **Drain** and **rinse** the black beans in a colander.
4. **Mix** all the salsa ingredients together (except the tortilla chips) in a bowl. **Season** well with salt and pepper.
5. **Spoon** the salsa into a bowl and **serve** with the tortilla chips on the side for dunking.

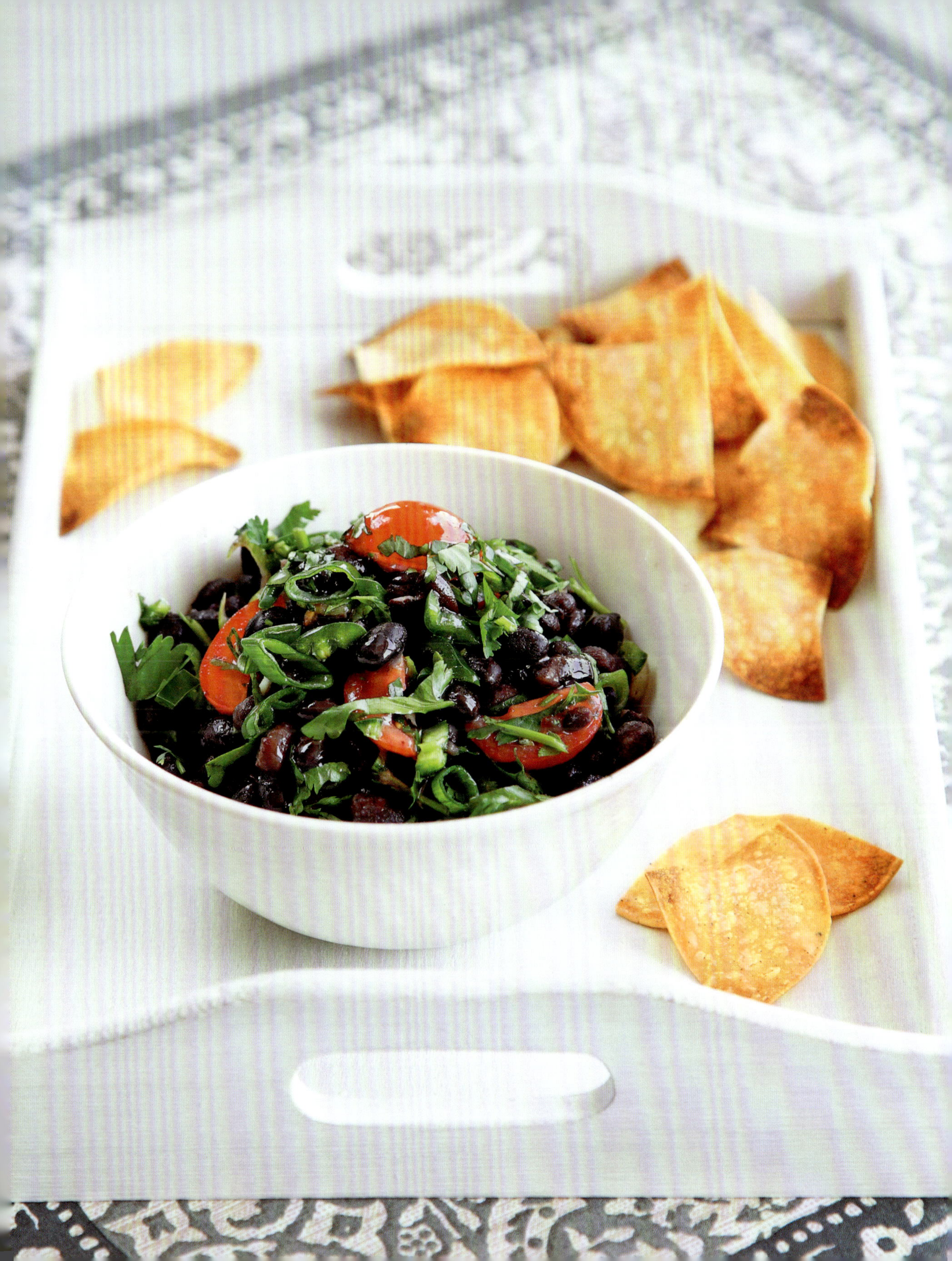

Serves 2–3 ▪ Preparation time: 10 minutes ▪ Cooking time: None
Total time: 10 minutes

Butter Bean & Anchovy Pâté

Ingredients

- 2 spring onions
- 40 g (1½ oz) fresh coriander
- 425 g (14 oz) can butter beans
- 50 g (2 oz) can anchovy fillets in oil
- 1 lemon
- 1 tablespoon olive oil
- pepper
- 4–6 slices of rye bread, to serve

Equipment

- kitchen scales
- 1 chopping board
- 1 sharp knife
- can opener
- 1 colander
- 1 lemon juicer
- measuring spoons
- 1 food processor or fork and bowl
- 1 mixing spoon

1. **Clear** your counter of clutter and **set out** all the equipment you need.
2. **Finely chop** the spring onions and then **chop** the coriander.
3. **Drain** and **rinse** the butter beans in a colander and **drain** the anchovies.
4. **Halve** and **juice** the lemon and **measure** out 2 tablespoons of juice.
5. **Place** all the ingredients, except the coriander pepper and rye bread, in a food processor and **blend** until well mixed but still rough in texture. Alternatively, **mash** the beans with a fork in a bowl, **finely chop** the anchovies and **mix** the ingredients together by hand.
6. **Stir** in the chopped coriander and **season** well with pepper.
7. **Toast** the rye bread.
8. **Spoon** the pâté into a serving bowl and **serve** with the toasted rye bread.

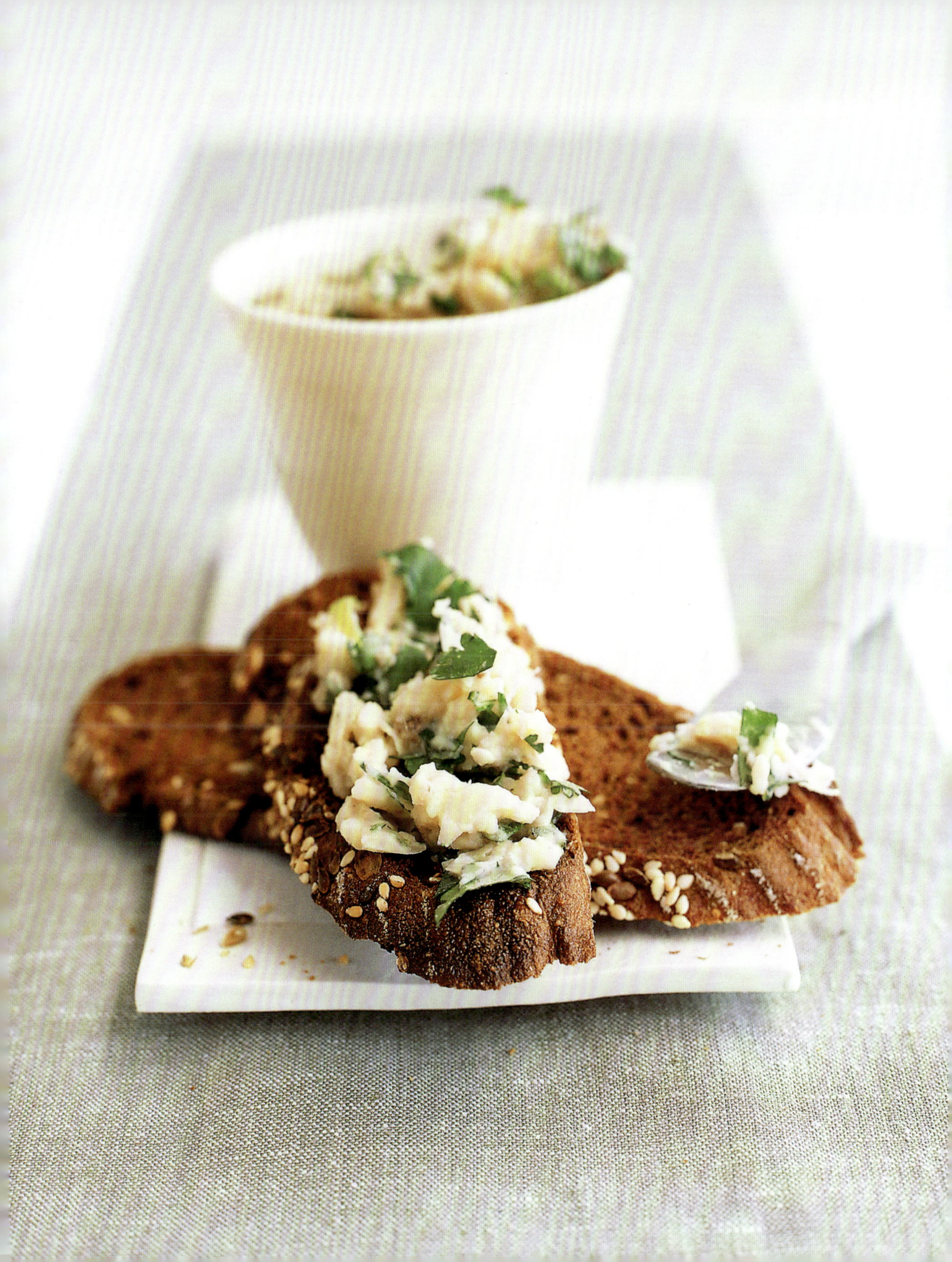

Serves 4 ▪ Preparation time: 10 minutes ▪ Cooking time: None
Total time: 10 minutes

Garlic & Bean Pâté

Ingredients

- **2 garlic cloves**
- **2 spring onions**
- **425 g (14 oz) can flageolet beans**
- **125 g (4 oz) cream cheese**
- **3 tablespoons basil pesto**
- **1 tablespoon olive oil**
- **salt and pepper**
- **½ cucumber, to serve**
- **4 pitta breads, to serve**

Equipment

- **kitchen scales**
- **1 chopping board**
- **1 sharp knife**
- **can opener**
- **1 colander**
- **measuring spoons**
- **1 food processor or blender**
- **2 spoons**
- **1 small mixing bowl**

1. **Clear** your counter of clutter and **set out** all the equipment you need.
2. **Chop** the garlic and spring onions.
3. **Drain** and **rinse** the flageolet beans in a colander.
4. **Put** the beans, cream cheese, garlic and 2 tablespoons of the pesto in a food processor or blender and **blend** until smooth.
5. **Add** the spring onions and salt and pepper to taste and blend for 10 seconds. **Spoon** the pâté into a serving dish and **chill** until required.
6. **Chop** the cucumber into batons.
7. **Lightly toast** the pitta breads, then **cut** them into thick strips.
8. **Mix** the remaining pesto with the olive oil and **drizzle** on top of the pâté. **Serve** with the cucumber and toasted pitta breads strips.

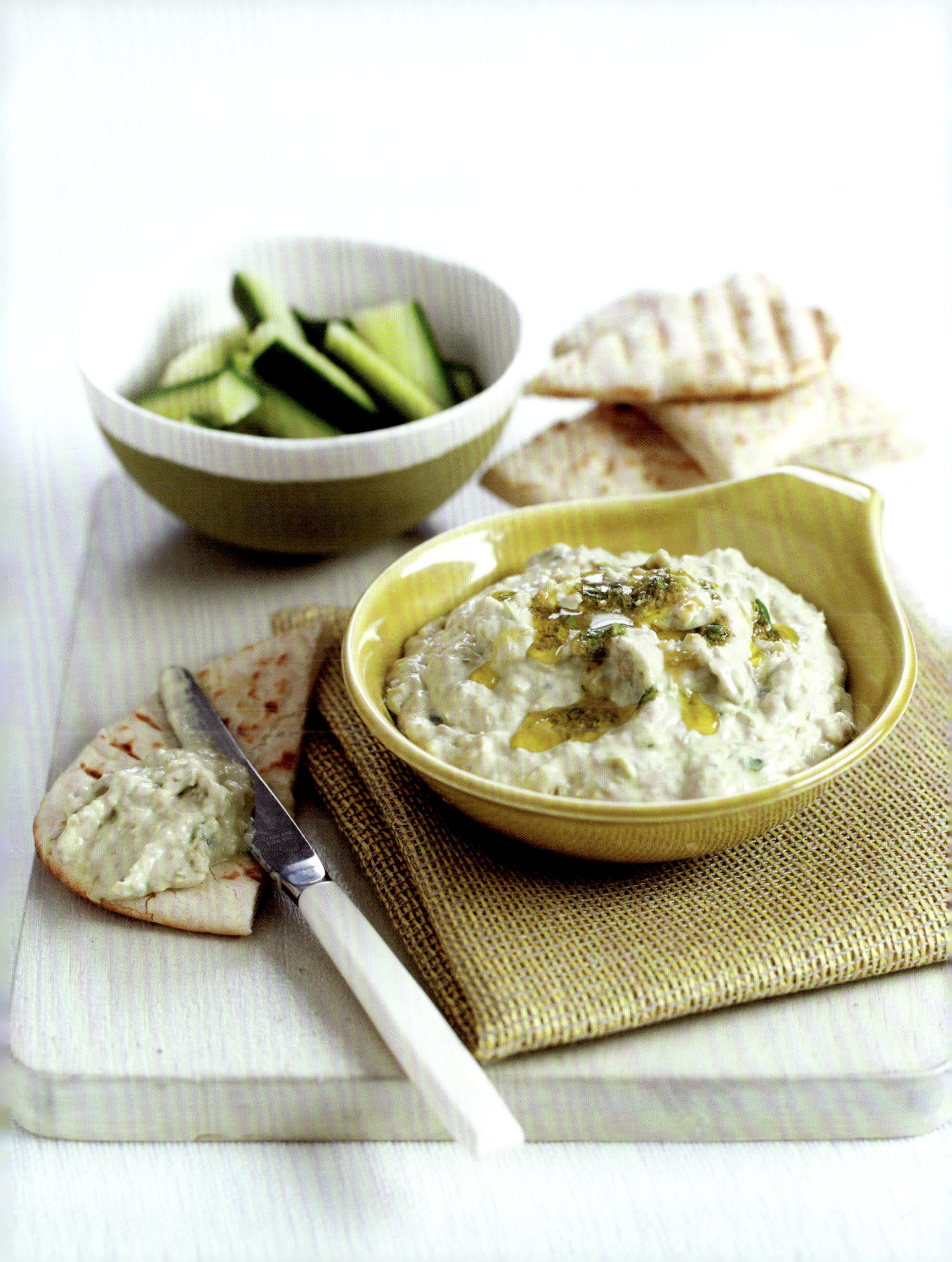

Serves 4 ▪ Preparation time: 10 minutes ▪ Cooking time: None
Total time: 10 minutes

Moroccan-style Hummus

Ingredients

- 1 garlic clove
- 400 g (13 oz) can chickpeas
- 1 tablespoon tahini paste
- 4 tablespoons Greek yogurt
- 1 tablespoon rose harissa paste, plus extra to drizzle
- 2 tablespoons lemon juice
- salt and pepper
- flatbreads, to serve

Equipment

- can opener
- 1 colander
- measuring spoons
- 1 food processor
- 1 spoon
- 1 spatula

TIP: Store in an airtight container in the refrigerator for up to 5 days for a quick snack option.

1. **Clear** your counter of clutter and **set out** all the equipment you need.
2. **Peel** the garlic. **Drain** and **rinse** the chickpeas in a colander.
3. **Place** all the ingredients (except the flatbreads) in a food processor, **reserving** a few chickpeas for garnish, and **blend** to a smooth paste. If the consistency is too thick, **add** 1 or 2 tablespoons of warm water.
4. **Season** to taste with salt and pepper, **transfer** the hummus to a serving bowl and **garnish** with the reserved chickpeas and a **drizzle** of extra harissa.
5. **Warm** the flatbreads in an oven on low or in a toaster.
6. **Serve** the hummus with the warmed flatbreads.

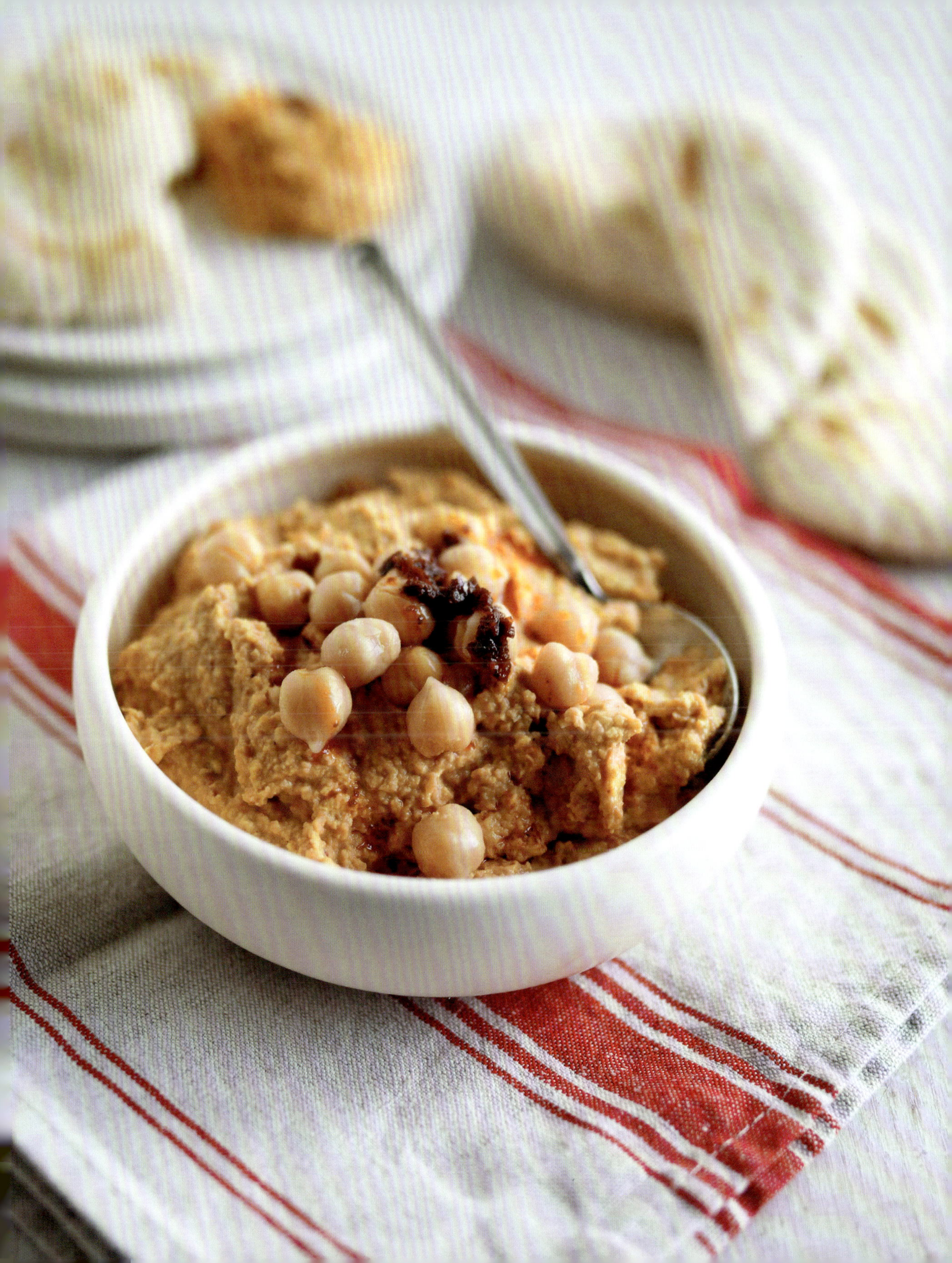

Serves 4 ▪ Preparation time: 15 minutes ▪ Cooking time: 2–3 minutes
Total time: 17–18 minutes

Roasted Peppers on Rye

Ingredients

- 175 g (6 oz) flame-roasted red peppers in brine or oil
- 2 tablespoons pine nuts
- 400 g (13 oz) can artichokes in water
- ½ lemon
- 125 g (4 oz) ricotta or cream cheese
- 8 small slices of seeded rye bread or multigrain bread
- 1 garlic clove
- 100 g (3½ oz) feta cheese (optional)
- salt and pepper

Equipment

- kitchen scales
- 1 chopping board
- 1 sharp knife
- 1 colander
- 1 frying pan
- 1 wooden spoon
- 1 food processor or blender
- 1 lemon juicer
- measuring spoons
- 1 spoon

1. **Clear** your counter of clutter and **set out** all the equipment you need.
2. **Drain** and **slice** the red peppers.
3. **Place** the pine nuts in a dry frying pan over a **medium-low heat** and **toast** for 2–3 minutes, **stirring** constantly with a wooden spoon, until they are golden brown. **Do not leave the pan unattended while the pine nuts are toasting, as they can burn easily.**
4. For the artichoke paste, **drain** the artichokes in a colander, **put** in a food processor or blender and **pulse** until roughly chopped and textured. **Juice** the lemon and **measure** out 1 tablespoon of juice. **Add** the ricotta or cream cheese and measured lemon juice and **pulse** to a paste. **Season** with salt and pepper.
5. **Toast** the bread.
6. **Peel** and **halve** the garlic clove and **rub** one side of the toast with the cut sides of the garlic clove.
7. **Spread** the artichoke paste over the garlic-rubbed toast and **top** with the red peppers. **Sprinkle** over the toasted pine nuts, **crumble** over the feta, if using, and **serve**.

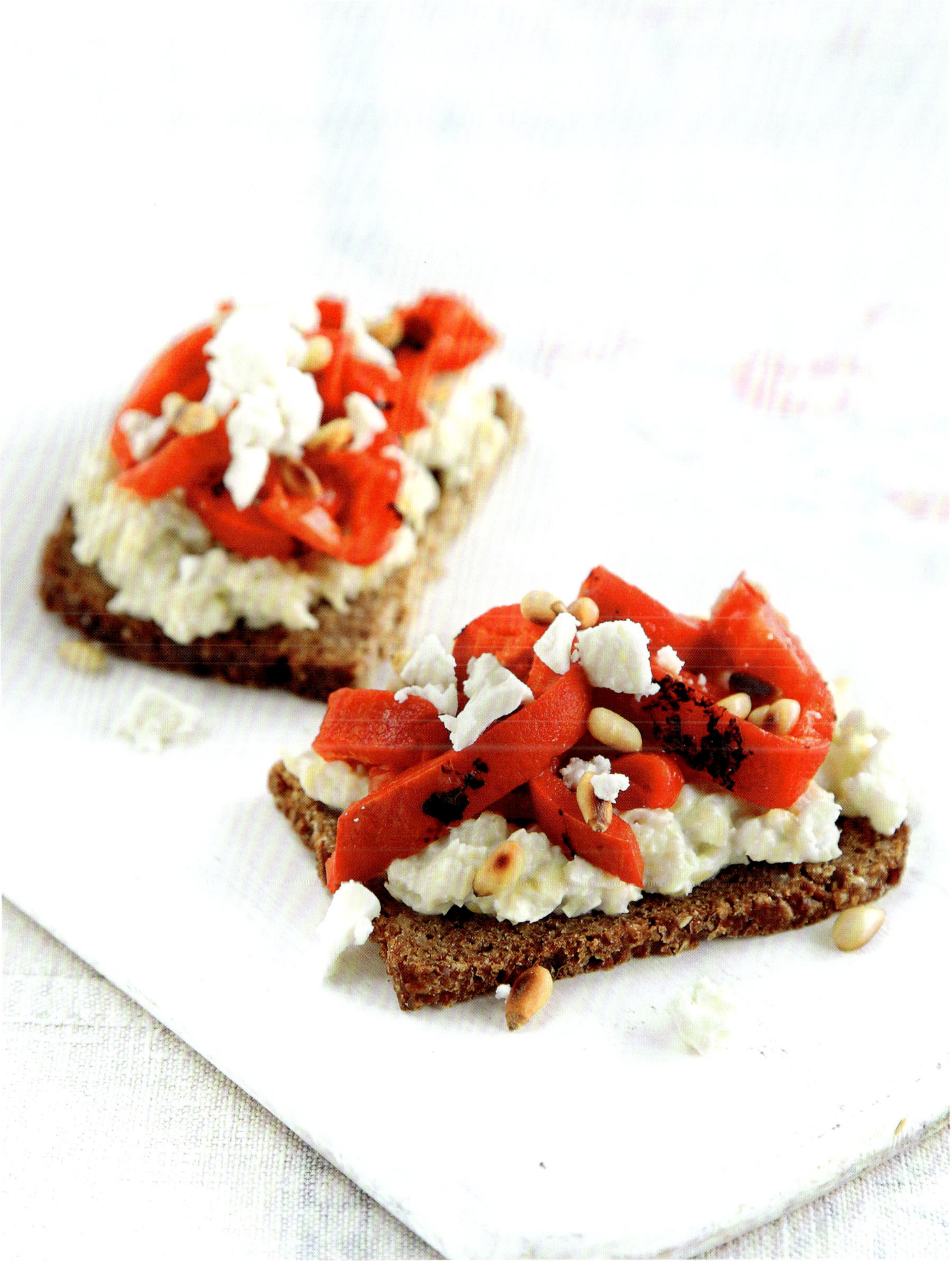

Makes about 25 ▪ Preparation time: 10–15 minutes ▪ Cooking time: 5–10 minutes
Total time: 15–25 minutes

Spicy Nut & Raisin Bites

Ingredients

- **450 g (14½ oz) blanched almonds**
- **200 g (7 oz) walnuts**
- **450 g (14½ oz) raisins**
- **120 g (4 oz) butter**
- **200 g (7 oz) clear honey**
- **1 teaspoon ras el hanout**
- **1 teaspoon ground cinnamon**
- **½ teaspoon ground ginger**
- **4 tablespoons sesame seeds**

Equipment

- **kitchen scales**
- **1 pestle and mortar or food processor**
- **1 heavy-based saucepan**
- **measuring spoons**
- **1 wooden spoon**
- **1 plate**

1. **Clear** your counter of clutter and **set out** all the equipment you need.
2. Using a pestle and mortar or a food processor, **pound** or **blend** the almonds, walnuts and raisins to a coarse paste.
3. **Melt** the butter in a heavy-based saucepan, **stir** in the honey and spices, then **add** the paste. **Stir** over a **low heat** until the mixture thickens and reaches a jam-like consistency. **Turn off** the heat and **leave to cool** completely.
4. Using wet fingertips, **divide** then **roll** about 25 small pieces of the mixture into truffle-sized balls. **Place** the sesame seeds on a plate. **Roll** the truffles in the seeds until evenly coated and **serve**.

Serves 2 ▪ Preparation time: 5 minutes ▪ Cooking time: None
Total time: 5 minutes

Balsamic & Black Pepper Strawberries

Ingredients

- **250g (8 oz) strawberries**
- **1 tablespoon balsamic vinegar**
- **½ teaspoon freshly ground black pepper**

Equipment

- **kitchen scales**
- **1 chopping board**
- **1 sharp knife**
- **1 mixing bowl**
- **measuring spoons**
- **1 mixing spoon**

1. **Clear** your counter of clutter and **set out** all the equipment you need.
2. **Hull** and **halve** the strawberries. **Place** in a mixing bowl and **pour** over the balsamic vinegar.
3. **Stir** well, to incorporate the flavours, then **add** the black pepper and **mix**. **Serve** immediately.

Serves 6 ▪ Preparation time: 10 minutes ▪ Cooking time: 17 minutes
Total time: 27 minutes

Roasted Almonds with Paprika

Ingredients

- 300 g (10 oz) blanched almonds
- 2 teaspoons olive oil
- 1 teaspoon sweet smoked paprika
- 1½ teaspoons sea salt flakes

Equipment

- kitchen scales
- 1 baking sheet
- measuring spoons
- 1 mixing spoon
- timer

1. **Clear** your counter of clutter and **set out** all the equipment you need.
2. **Preheat** the oven to **180°C (350°F), Gas Mark 4**.
3. **Place** the almonds on a baking sheet and **roast** in the oven for 15 minutes until starting to brown. **Set a timer** so you don't forget.
4. **Stir** through the remaining ingredients, **return** to the oven and **cook** for a further 2 minutes until heated through. **Leave to cool**, then **serve**.

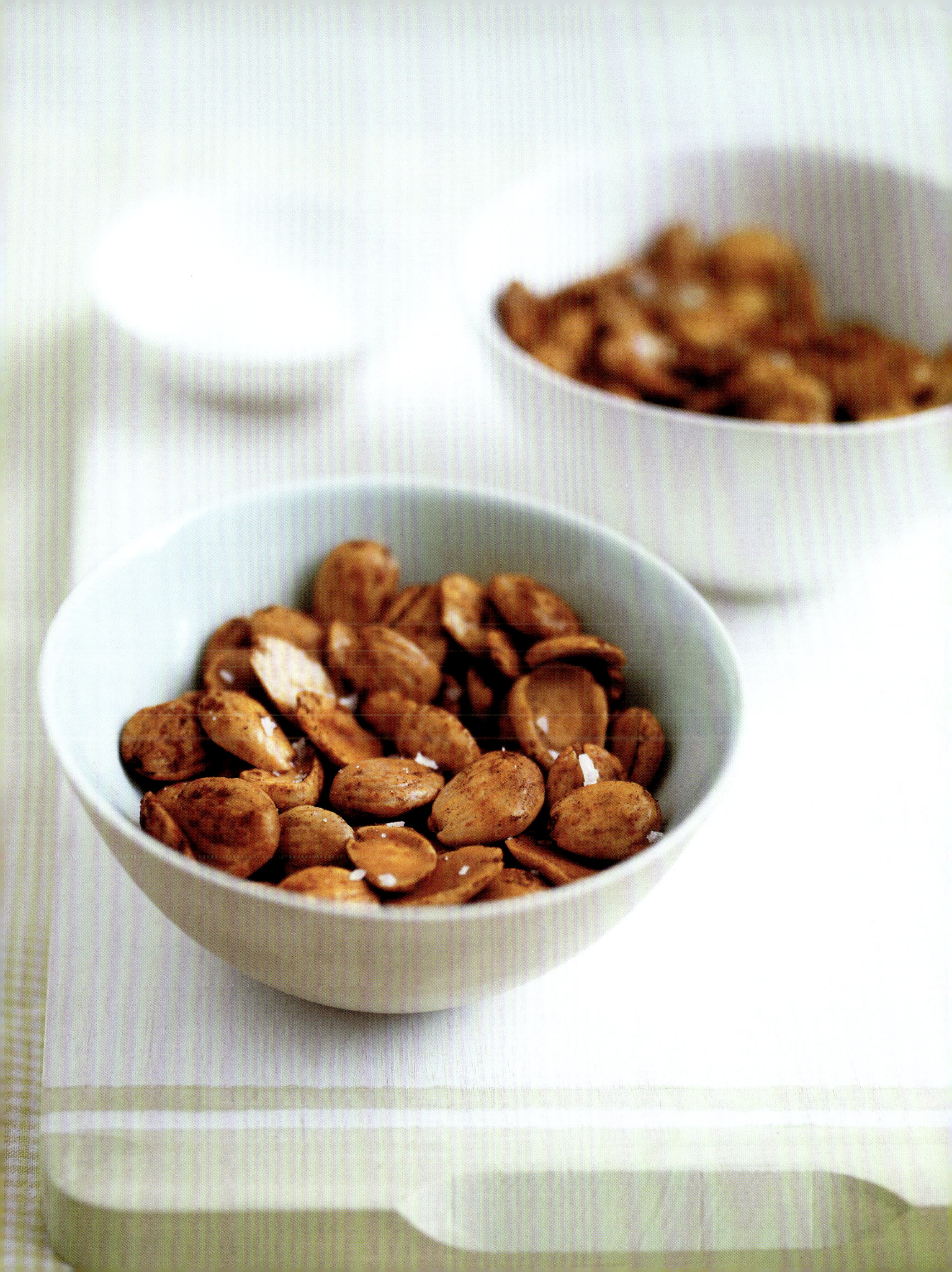

Makes 12–15 ▪ Preparation time: 5 minutes ▪ Cooking time: 5–7 minutes
Total time: 10–12 minutes

Cheese & Chive Crisps

Ingredients

- 75 g (3 oz) Parmesan cheese
- 20 g (¾ oz) fresh chives or 2 teaspoons dried chives
- freshly ground black pepper

Equipment

- kitchen scales
- 1 large baking sheet
- nonstick baking paper
- 1 grater
- 1 chopping board
- 1 sharp knife
- 1 small mixing bowl
- 1 mixing spoon
- 9 cm (3½ inch) plain cutter
- 1 tablespoon
- 1 wire rack
- 1 spatula

1. **Clear** your counter of clutter and **set out** all the equipment you need.
2. **Preheat** the oven to **200°C (400°F), Gas Mark 6**. **Line** a baking sheet with nonstick baking paper.
3. **Finely grate** the Parmesan. If using fresh chives, **finely chop**.
4. **Mix** the Parmesan and chives (either fresh or dried) together with a generous pinch of black pepper in a small mixing bowl.
5. **Place** the cutter on the prepared baking sheet and evenly **sprinkle** 1 rounded tablespoon of the mixture inside. **Remove** the cutter and **repeat** with the remaining mixture to make 12–15 crisps.
6. **Bake** in the oven for 5–7 minutes until golden. Carefully **transfer** to a wire rack to cool and crisp before **serving**.

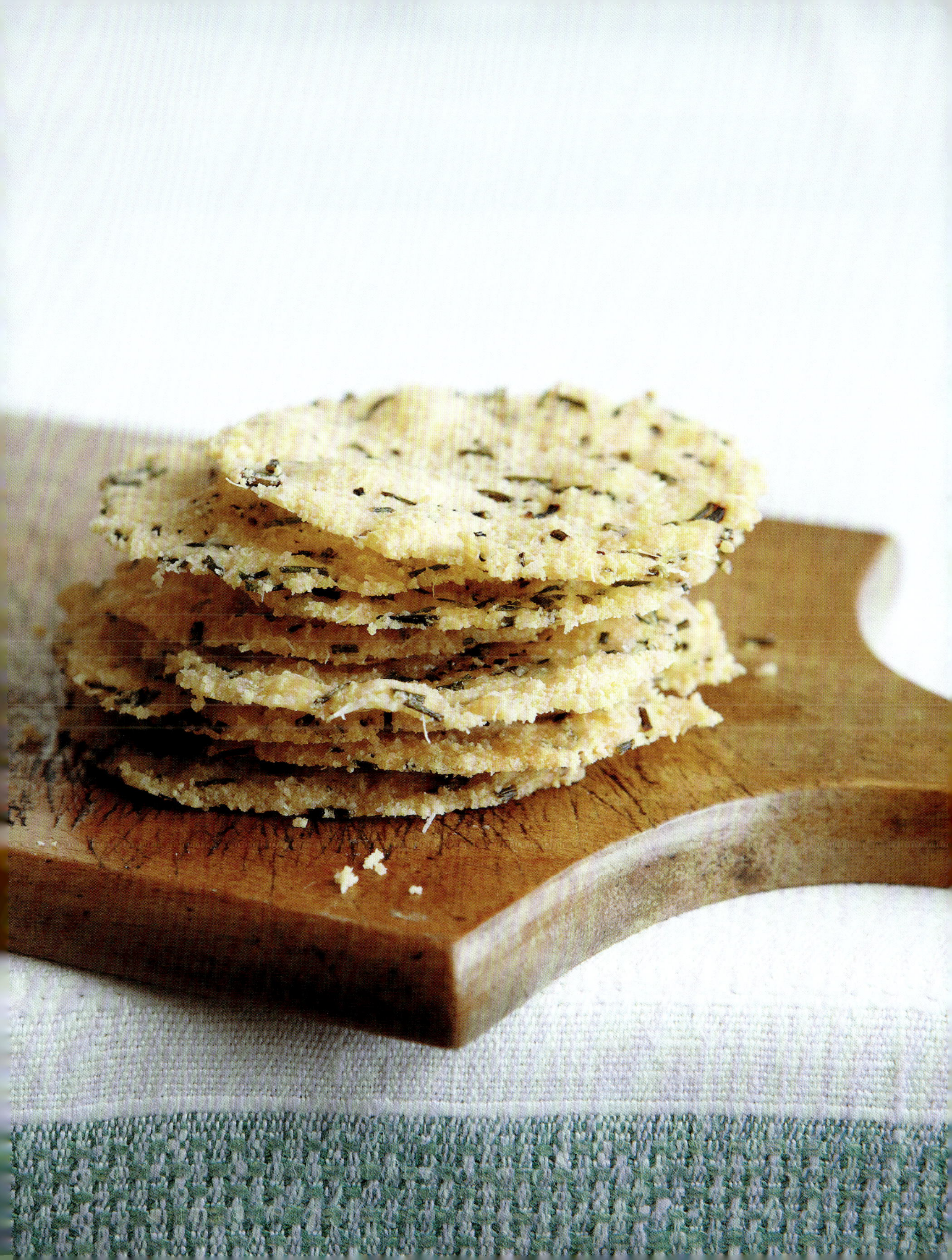

Serves 2–3 ▪ Preparation time: 5–10 minutes ▪ Cooking time: None
Total time: 5–10 minutes

Banana & Oat Smoothie

Ingredients

- **1 small banana**
- **1 tablespoon pomegranate juice**
- **300 ml (½ pint) soya milk**
- **1 tablespoon almonds**
- **1 tablespoon rolled oats**
- **½ teaspoon clear honey**
- **½ tablespoon ground flaxseeds**
- **2 tablespoons natural yogurt**

Equipment

- **1 measuring jug**
- **1 chopping board**
- **1 sharp knife**
- **1 blender**
- **measuring spoons**

1. **Clear** your counter of clutter and **set out** all the equipment you need.
2. **Peel** and **roughly chop** the banana.
3. **Place** all the ingredients in a blender and **blend** until smooth and creamy.
4. **Pour** into 2 or 3 glasses and **serve** immediately.

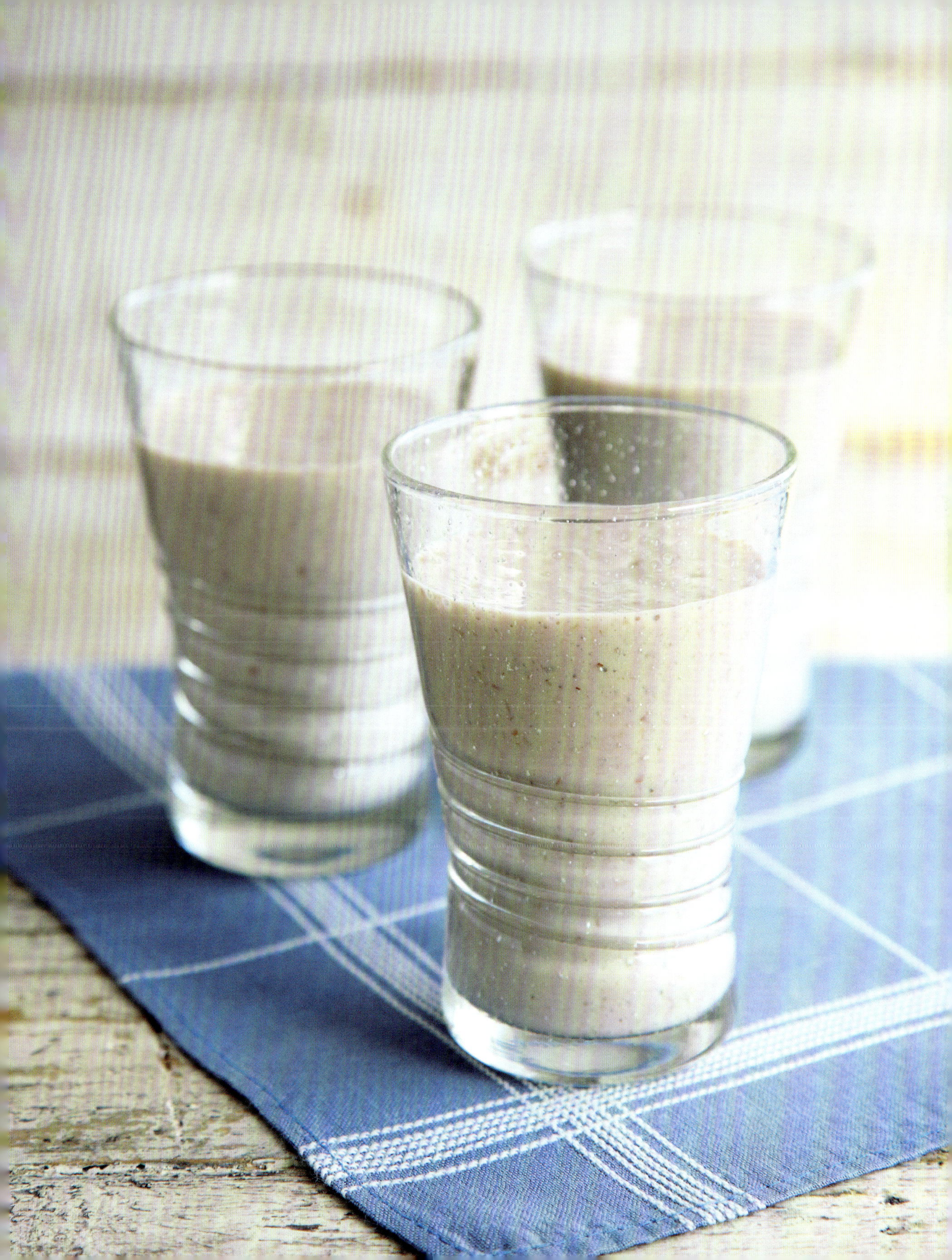

Serves 4 · Preparation time: 5–10 minutes · Cooking time: None
Total time: 5–10 minutes

Yogurt & Berry Smoothie

Ingredients

- 500 g (1 lb) fresh or frozen mixed summer berries, defrosted if frozen, plus a few extra to decorate
- 300 ml (½ pint) natural yogurt
- 4 tablespoons millet flakes
- 3 tablespoons clear honey
- 300 ml (½ pint) cranberry juice

Equipment

- kitchen scales
- measuring jugs
- measuring spoons
- 1 food processor or blender

1. **Clear** your counter of clutter and **set out** all the equipment you need.
2. If using frozen berries, **defrost** them in the microwave for 1–2 minutes.
3. **Place** all the ingredients in a food processor or a blender and **blitz** until smooth.
4. **Pour** into 4 glasses, **decorate** with a few extra whole frozen berries and **serve** immediately.

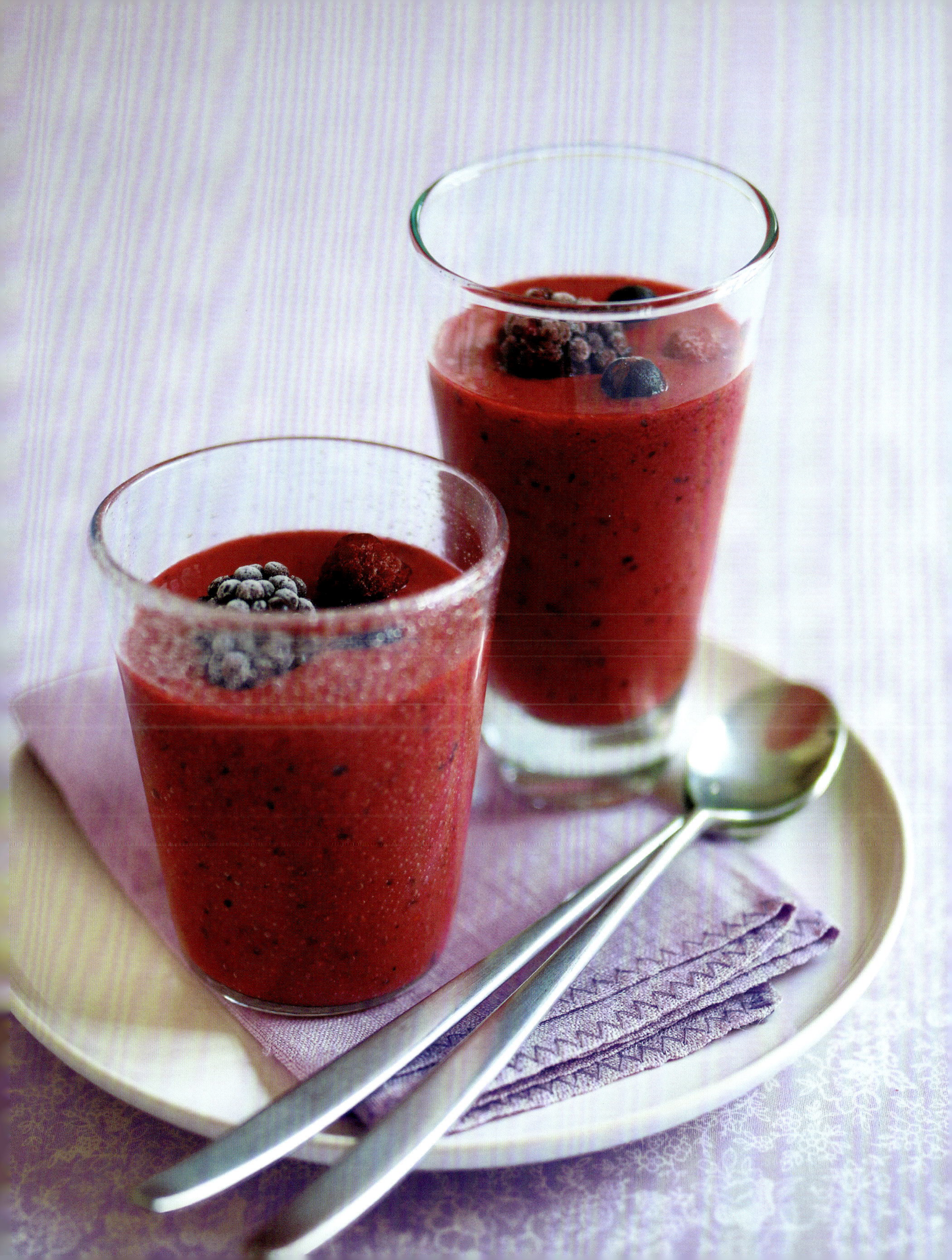

Serves 4 ▪ Preparation time: 10 minutes ▪ Cooking time: None
Total time: 10 minutes

Creamy Mango Smoothie

Ingredients

- **2 ripe mangoes**
- **1 banana**
- **2 tablespoons natural yogurt**
- **500 ml (17 fl oz) soya milk**
- **clear honey, to sweeten (optional)**
- **ice cubes, to serve**

Equipment

- **1 measuring jug**
- **1 chopping board**
- **1 vegetable peeler**
- **1 sharp knife**
- **1 blender**
- **1 tablespoon**

1. **Clear** your counter of clutter and **set out** all the equipment you need.
2. **Peel** and **stone** the mangoes. **Peel** and **roughly chop** the banana.
3. **Place** all the ingredients, except the honey and ice, in a blender and **blend** until smooth.
4. **Taste** for sweetness and **add** honey, if required, then **blend** again.
5. **Pour** into 4 tall glasses and **serve** with ice cubes.

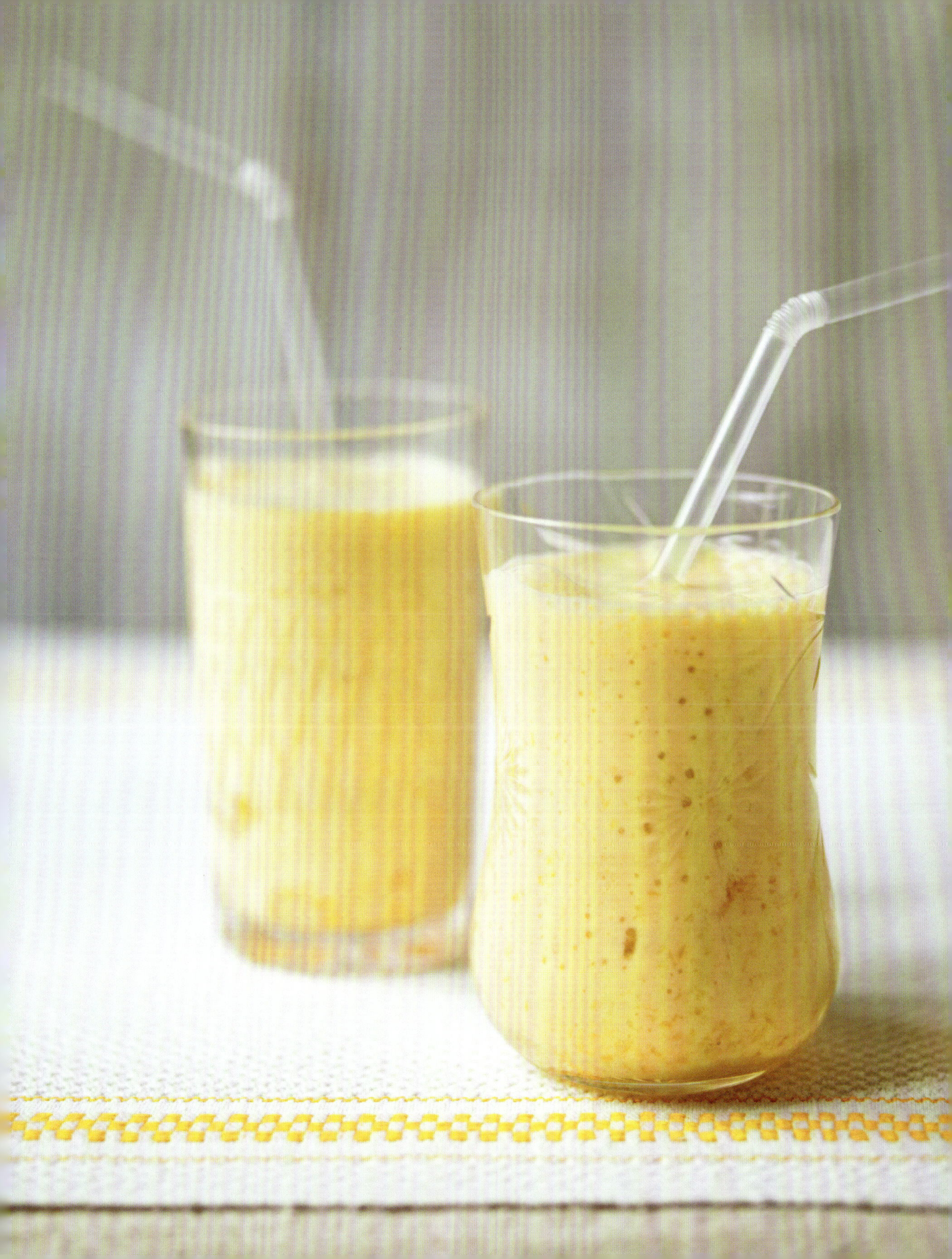

Lunch

Serves 4 ▪ Preparation time: 10 minutes ▪ Cooking time: None
Total time: 10 minutes

Lentil & Goats' Cheese Salad

Ingredients

- 125 g (4 oz) roasted red and yellow peppers in brine or oil
- 400 g (13 oz) can Puy lentils in water
- 125 g (4 oz) baby spinach
- 50 g (2 oz) walnut pieces
- 2 tablespoons balsamic vinegar
- 3 tablespoons walnut oil
- 1 teaspoon Dijon mustard
- 125 g (4 oz) fresh goats' cheese
- salt and pepper
- crusty bread, to serve

Equipment

- kitchen scales
- 1 chopping board
- 1 sharp knife
- can opener
- 1 sieve
- 1 mixing bowl
- 1 mixing spoon
- 1 small bowl
- measuring spoons
- 1 fork or whisk

1. **Clear** your counter of clutter and **set out** all the equipment you need.
2. **Drain** and **chop** the red and yellow peppers. **Drain** and **rinse** the lentils.
3. **Place** the spinach, lentils, peppers and walnut pieces in a mixing bowl and **mix** gently.
4. For the dressing, **whisk** together the balsamic vinegar, walnut oil and Dijon mustard in a small bowl and **season** to taste with salt and pepper. **Pour** over the lentil mixture and **toss** lightly to combine.
5. **Divide** the salad between 4 bowls and roughly **crumble** over the goats' cheese. **Serve** with crusty bread.

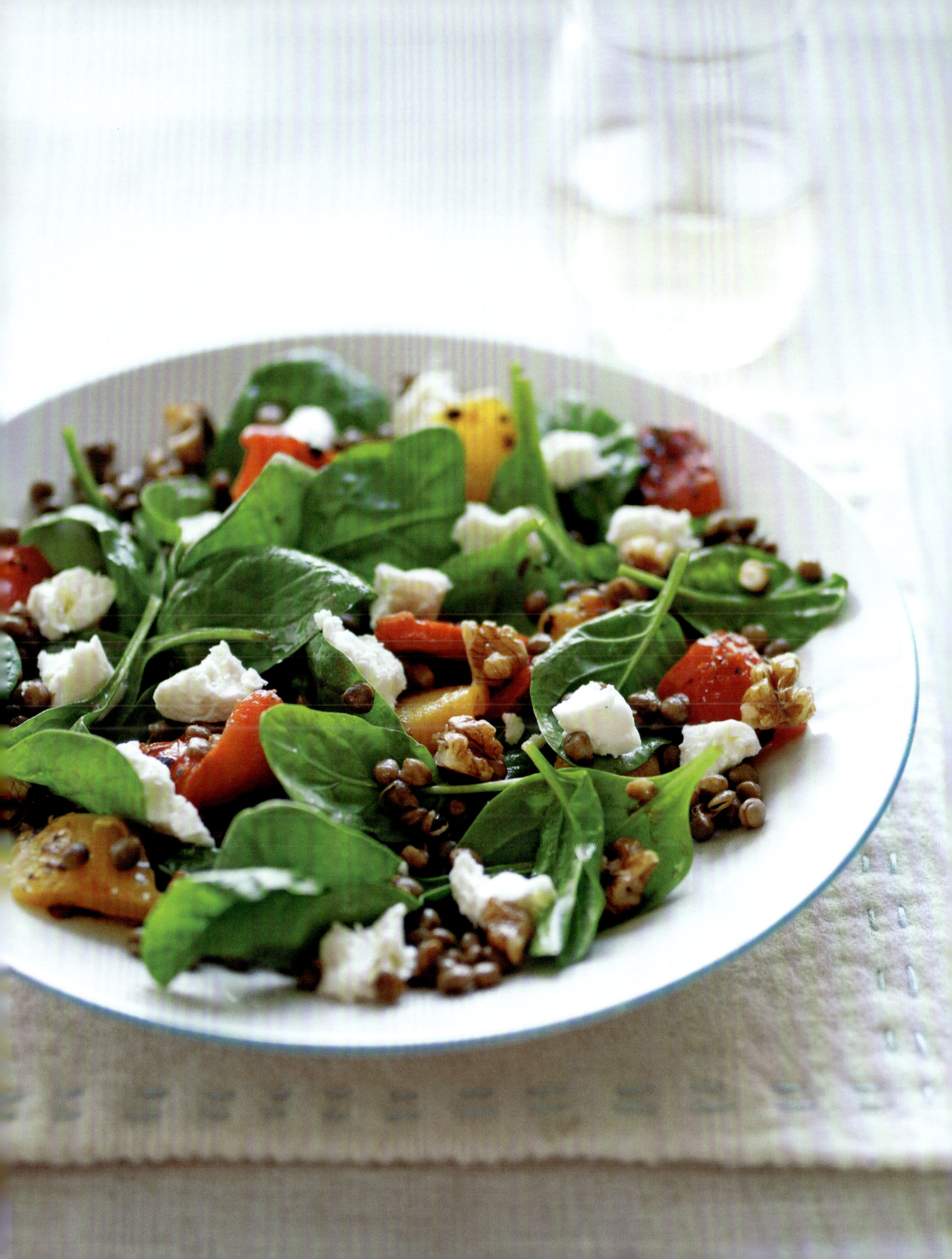

Serves 4 ▪ Preparation time: 5–10 minutes ▪ Cooking time: 10 minutes
Total time: 15–20 minutes

Chicken & Noodle Miso Soup

Ingredients

- **900 ml (1½ pints) hot chicken stock**
- **4 spring onions**
- **1 carrot**
- **4 baby pak choi**
- **200 g (7 oz) ready-cooked chicken breast**
- **2 × 18 g (¾ oz) sachets miso soup paste or 2 tablespoons miso paste**
- **2 teaspoons ready-chopped ginger**
- **300 g (10 oz) ready-cooked medium egg noodles**

Equipment

- **kitchen scales**
- **1 measuring jug**
- **1 chopping board**
- **1 sharp knife**
- **1 medium saucepan**
- **1 wooden spoon**
- **measuring spoons**

1. **Clear** your counter of clutter and **set out** all the equipment you need.
2. **Prepare** the chicken stock according to the packet instructions.
3. **Cut** the spring onions and carrot into thin strips. **Halve** the pak choi. **Slice** the chicken breast into strips.
4. **Place** the chicken stock, miso paste and ginger in a medium saucepan and bring to the **boil**. **Simmer** for 2 minutes.
5. **Add** the spring onions, carrot, pak choi and chicken and **simmer** for 3–4 minutes more.
6. **Stir** in the noodles and **cook** for a further 2 minutes to heat through. **Divide** between 4 bowls and **serve** immediately.

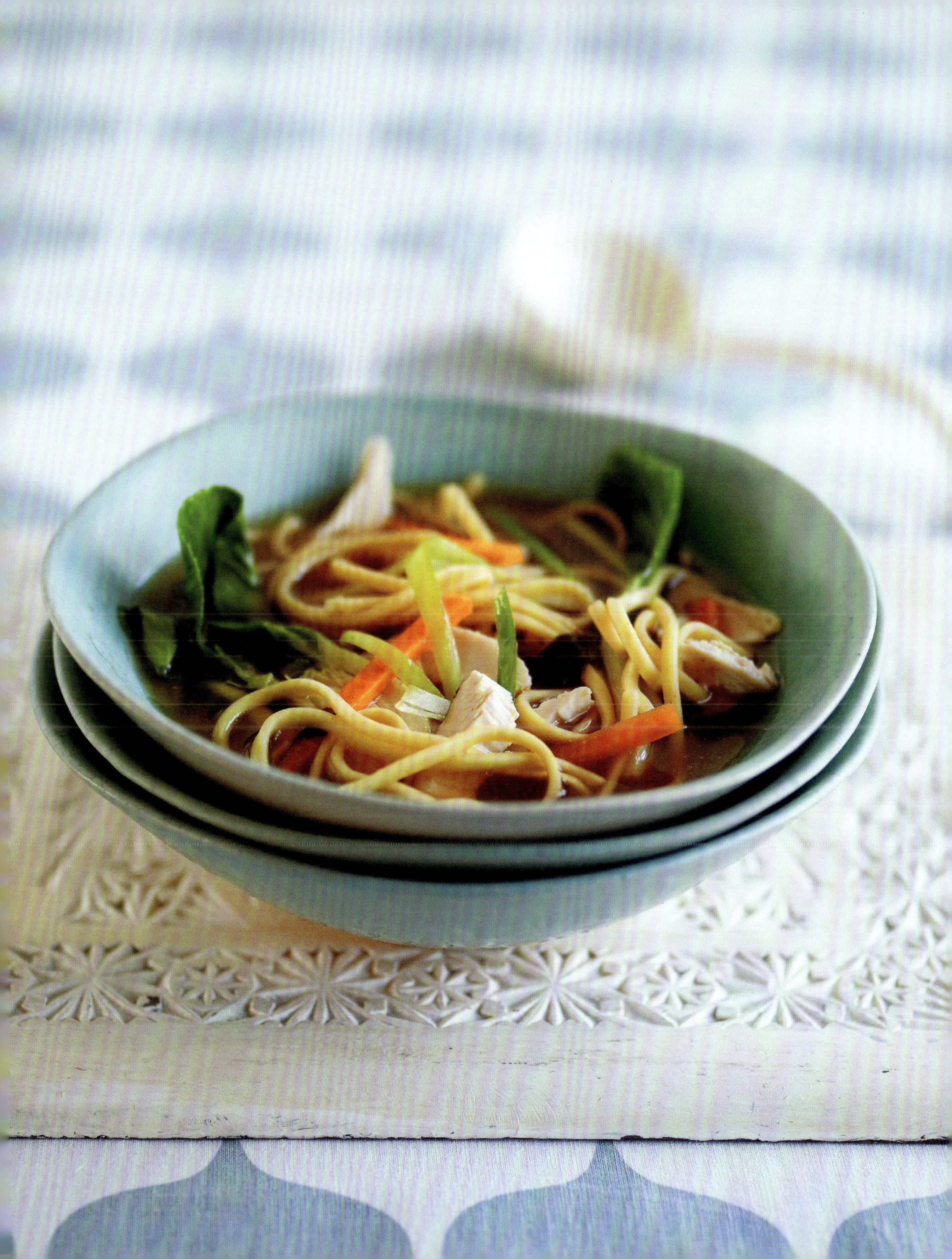

Serves 4 ▪ Preparation time: 15 minutes ▪ Cooking time: None
Total time: 15 minutes

Chopped Salad

Ingredients

- **1 iceberg lettuce**
- **1 ripe avocado**
- **2 ripe tomatoes**
- **½ red onion**
- **10 g (¼ oz) fresh coriander leaves**
- **1 jalapeño chilli (optional)**
- **400 g (13 oz) can red kidney beans**
- **1½ limes**
- **3 tablespoons olive oil**
- **corn chips, to garnish**
- **soured cream, to serve (optional)**

Equipment

- **kitchen scales**
- **1 chopping board**
- **1 sharp knife**
- **can opener**
- **1 colander**
- **1 large salad bowl**
- **1 mixing spoon**
- **1 lemon juicer**
- **1 small bowl**
- **measuring spoons**
- **1 fork or whisk**

1. **Clear** your counter of clutter and **set out** all the equipment you need.
2. **Cut** the lettuce into bite-sized pieces. **Peel, stone** and **dice** the avocado. **Chop** the tomatoes. **Finely dice** the red onion. **Chop** the coriander leaves and **finely slice** the jalapeño chilli, if using.
3. **Drain** and **rinse** the kidney beans in a colander.
4. **Put** the lettuce into a large salad bowl. **Add** the beans, avocado, tomatoes and red onion with the coriander and chilli, if using. **Mix** all the ingredients together.
5. Then make the dressing. **Halve** and **juice** the limes, then **whisk** together with the oil in a small bowl. **Drizzle** the dressing over the salad and **mix** lightly to combine.
6. **Garnish** with lightly crushed corn chips and **serve** with soured cream, if liked.

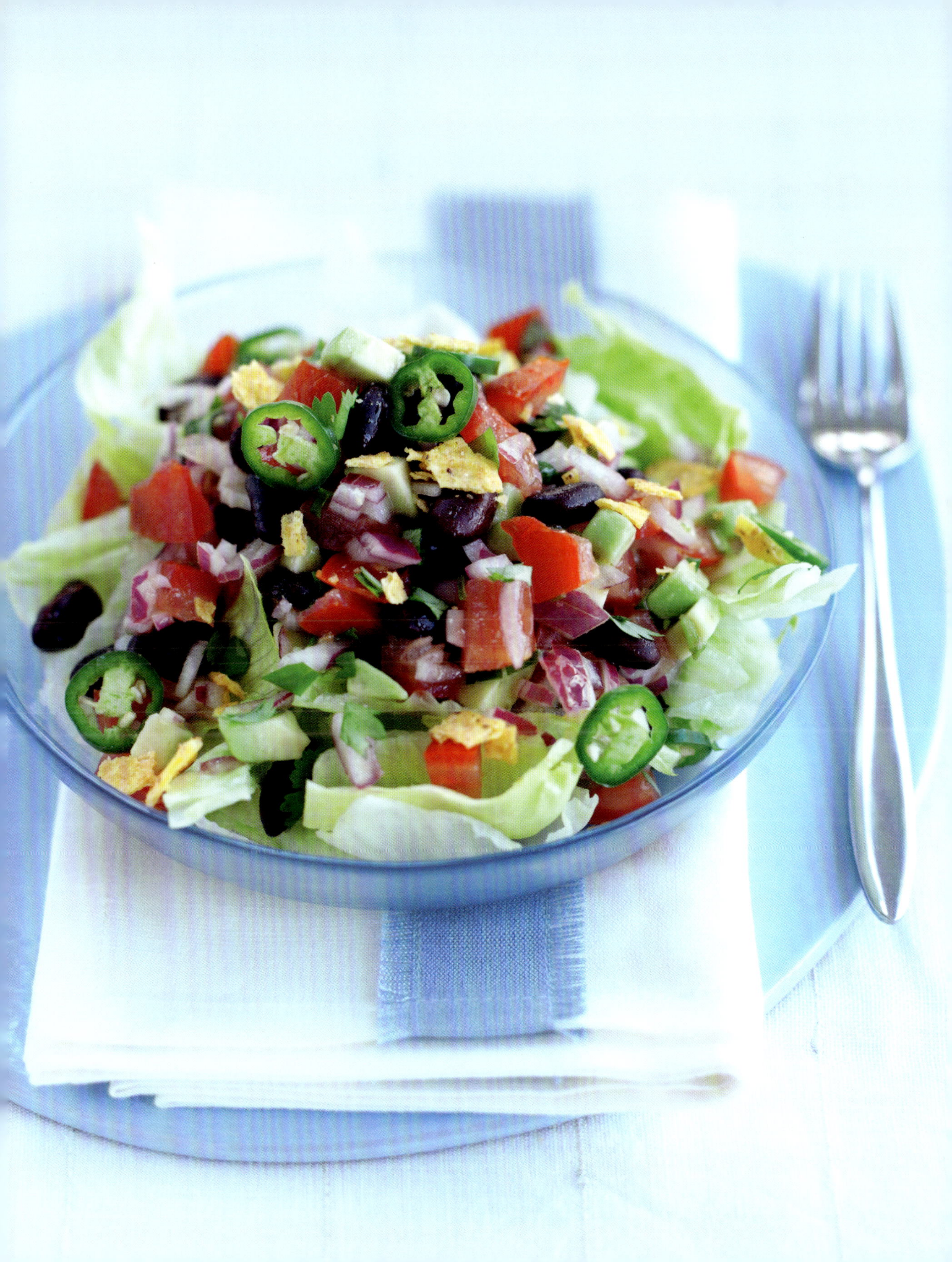

Serves 2 · Preparation time: 15 minutes · Cooking time: 4–6 minutes
Total time: 19–21 minutes

Griddled Greek-style Sandwiches

Ingredients

- ¼ small red onion
- 8 cherry tomatoes
- 4 pitted black olives
- 5 cm (2 inch) piece of cucumber
- 1 teaspoon dried oregano
- 50 g (2 oz) feta cheese
- ½ lemon
- 25 g (1 oz) Cheddar cheese
- 2 round seeded pitta breads
- olive oil, for brushing
- pepper

Equipment

- kitchen scales
- 1 chopping board
- 1 sharp knife
- 1 small bowl
- 1 mixing spoon
- 1 lemon juicer
- measuring spoons
- 1 grater
- 1 pastry brush
- 1 griddle pan
- 1 spatula

1. **Clear** your counter of clutter and **set out** all the equipment you need.
2. **Thinly slice** the red onion. **Quarter** the tomatoes. **Chop** the black olives. **Deseed** the cucumber and **cut** into small pieces.
3. **Add** the red onion, tomatoes, olives, cucumber and oregano to a small bowl and **crumble** in the feta. **Mix** together. **Juice** the lemon and **add** 1 teaspoon of juice to the mixture, **season** to taste with pepper and gently **mix**.
4. **Grate** the Cheddar.
5. **Split** each pitta bread in half horizontally. **Divide** the feta mixture between the bottom halves of the pitta breads, then **add** the Cheddar. **Cover** with the top halves of the pitta breads.
6. **Brush** a griddle pan with oil and **heat** over a **medium heat**. When hot, **add** the sandwiches, **press down** gently with a spatula and **cook** for 2–3 minutes on each side until golden and the cheese has melted. **Serve** immediately.

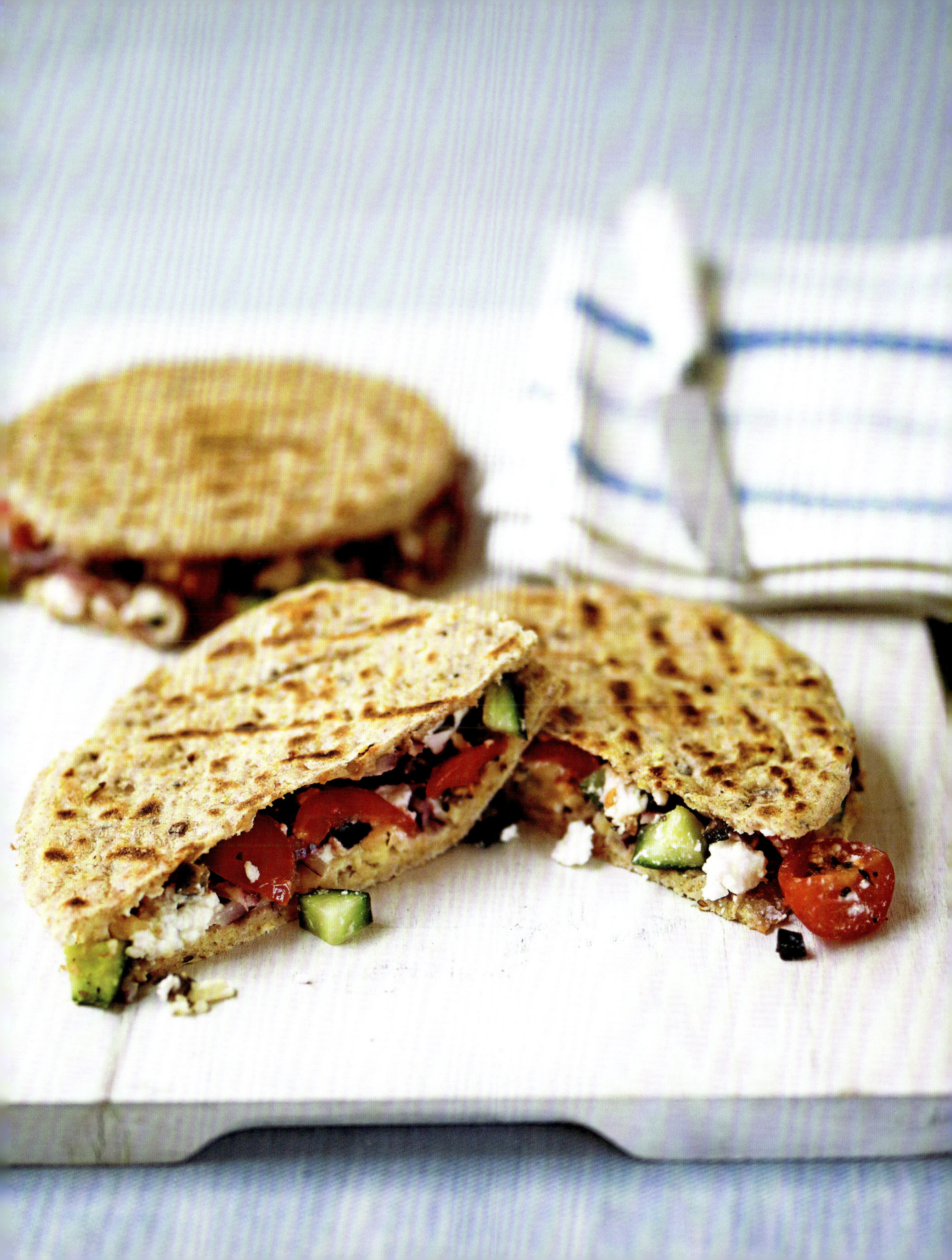

Serves 4–6 ▪ Preparation time: 10 minutes ▪ Cooking time: None
Total time: 10 minutes

Fig, Raspberry & Prosciutto Salad

Ingredients

- **6 ripe figs**
- **150 g (5 oz) rocket and beetroot salad mix**
- **150 g (5 oz) fresh raspberries**
- **8 slices of prosciutto**
- **2 tablespoons aged balsamic vinegar**
- **2 tablespoons olive oil**
- **2 large buffalo mozzarella balls, each about 150 g (5 oz)**

Equipment

- **kitchen scales**
- **1 chopping board**
- **1 sharp knife**
- **1 large bowl**
- **1 spoon**
- **1 large serving plate**
- **measuring spoons**
- **1 small bowl**
- **1 fork or whisk**

1. **Clear** your counter of clutter and **set out** all the equipment you need.
2. **Halve** the figs.
3. **Put** the rocket and beetroot salad in a large bowl, **add** the halved figs, the raspberries and the prosciutto, **toss** carefully and **transfer** to a large serving plate.
4. Make the dressing by **whisking** together the balsamic vinegar and oil in a small bowl.
5. **Drain**, then **tear** each mozzarella ball into 3 pieces and **arrange** them on the salad. **Drizzle** the dressing over the salad and **serve**.

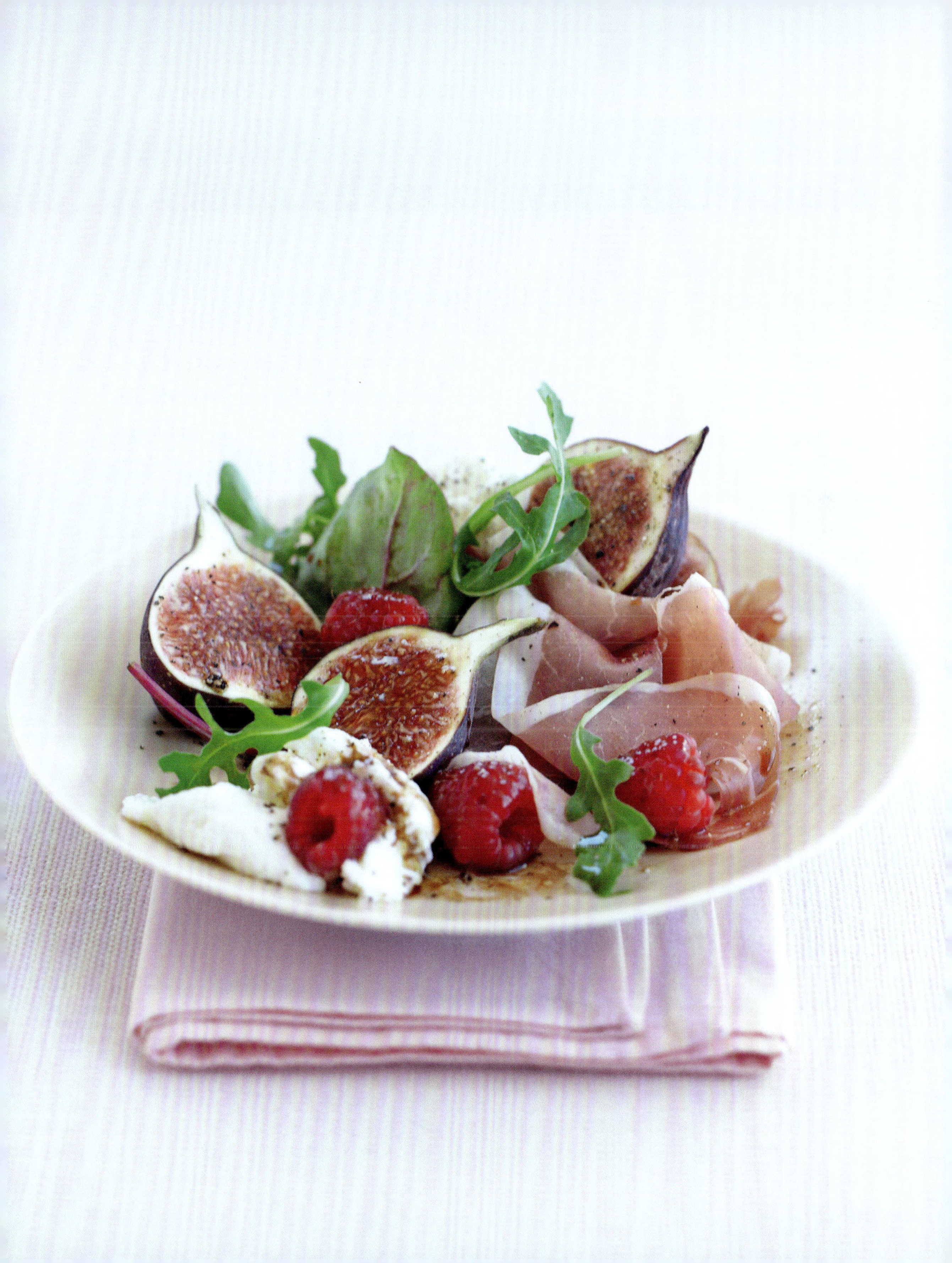

Serves 4 ▪ Preparation 5–10 minutes ▪ Cooking time: 10–12 minutes
Total time: 15–22 minutes

Quick Garlicky Tomato Lentils

Ingredients

- **1 large onion**
- **2 garlic cloves**
- **2 x 390 g (12½ oz) cans green lentils**
- **2 tablespoons olive or vegetable oil**
- **440 g (14¼ oz) jar tomato-based pasta sauce**
- **1 teaspoon dried oregano or mixed herbs (optional)**
- **100 g (3½ oz) Cheddar cheese, Parmesan cheese or other hard Italian cheese (optional)**
- **crusty bread, to serve**

Equipment

- **kitchen scales**
- **1 chopping board**
- **1 sharp knife**
- **can opener**
- **1 sieve**
- **1 large frying pan**
- **measuring spoons**
- **1 wooden spoon**
- **1 grater**

1. **Clear** your counter of clutter and **set out** all the equipment you need.
2. **Chop** the onion and garlic.
3. **Drain** and **rinse** the lentils.
4. **Heat** the oil in a large frying pan and **cook** the onion and garlic over a **medium heat** for 6–7 minutes, **stirring** frequently, until softened.
5. **Add** the pasta sauce, dried oregano or mixed herbs, if using, and the lentils and **heat** to simmering point.
6. **Grate** the cheese, if using.
7. **Spoon** the lentil mixture into bowls. **Scatter** with the cheese, if using, and **serve** immediately with crusty bread.

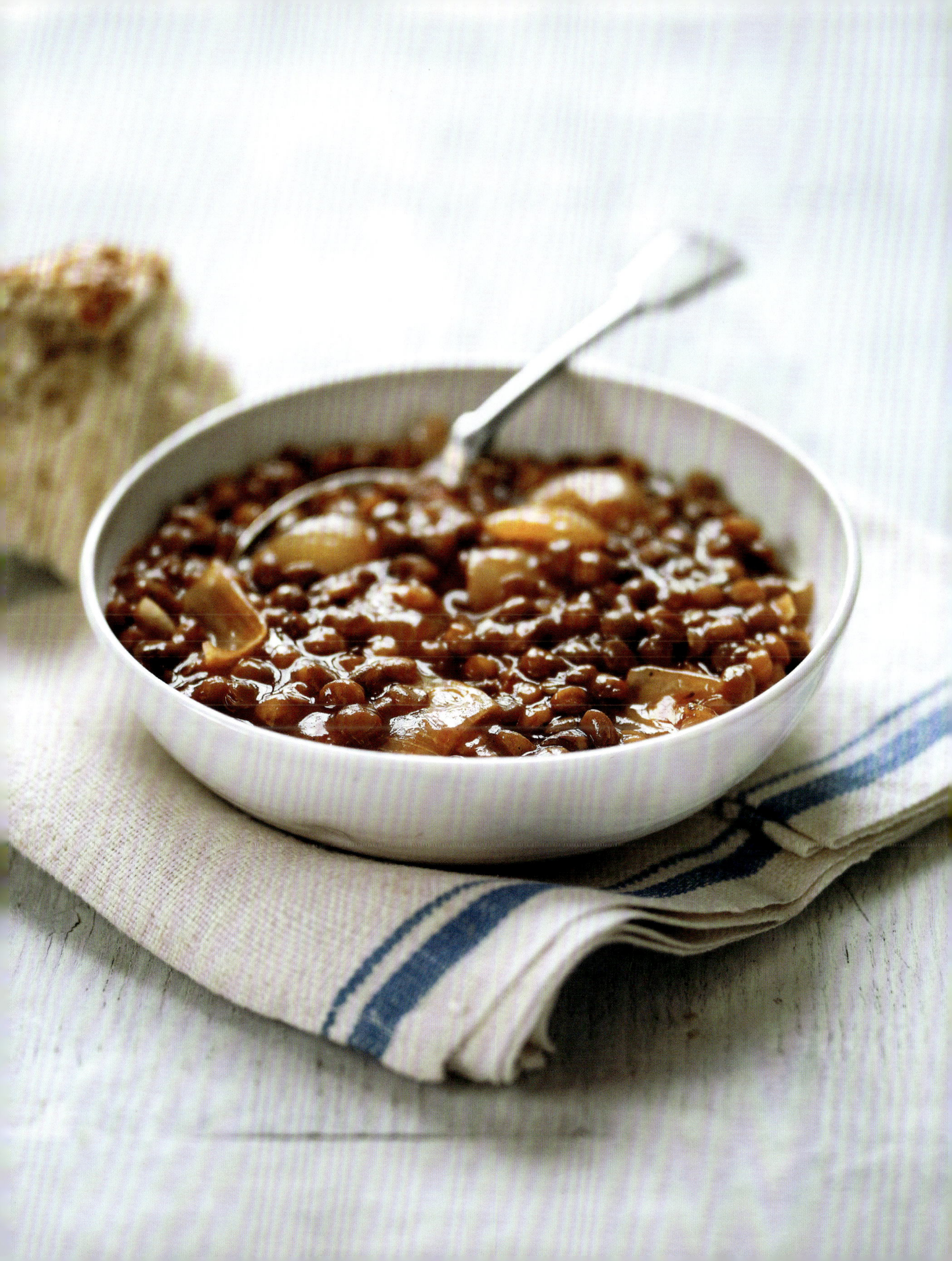

Serves 4 ▪ Preparation time: 15 minutes ▪ Cooking time: 1–2 minutes
Total time: 16–17 minutes

Smoked Chicken Salad

Ingredients

- 2 red onions
- 150 g (5 oz) cherry tomatoes
- 300 g (10 oz) skinless smoked (cooked) chicken breast
- 50 g (2 oz) pumpkin seeds
- 1 ripe avocado
- 1 lime
- 1 tablespoon Dijon mustard
- 75 g (3 oz) mixed salad leaves
- salt and pepper
- small handful of fresh basil and/or flat leaf parsley leaves, to garnish (optional)

Equipment

- kitchen scales
- 1 chopping board
- 1 sharp knife
- 1 sieve
- 1 small frying pan
- 1 wooden spoon
- 1 lemon juicer
- measuring spoons
- 1 food processor
- 1 salad bowl
- salad servers

1. **Clear** your counter of clutter and **set out** all the equipment you need.
2. **Finely slice** the red onions and **rinse** in water using a sieve. **Halve** the cherry tomatoes.
3. **Shred** the smoked chicken.
4. **Heat** a small frying pan until hot, **add** the pumpkin seeds and **dry-fry** over a **high heat** for 1–2 minutes, **stirring** occasionally, until golden.
5. To make the dressing, **peel**, **stone** and **roughly chop** the avocado. **Halve** and **juice** the lime and **measure** out 2 tablespoons of juice. **Place** the avocado, measured lime juice and Dijon mustard in a food processor and **blend** until smooth. **Season** to taste with salt and pepper.
6. **Place** the chicken, red onions, tomatoes, pumpkin seeds and salad leaves in a salad bowl and **toss** together. **Drizzle** over the dressing, **garnish** with basil and parsley leaves, if liked, and **serve**.

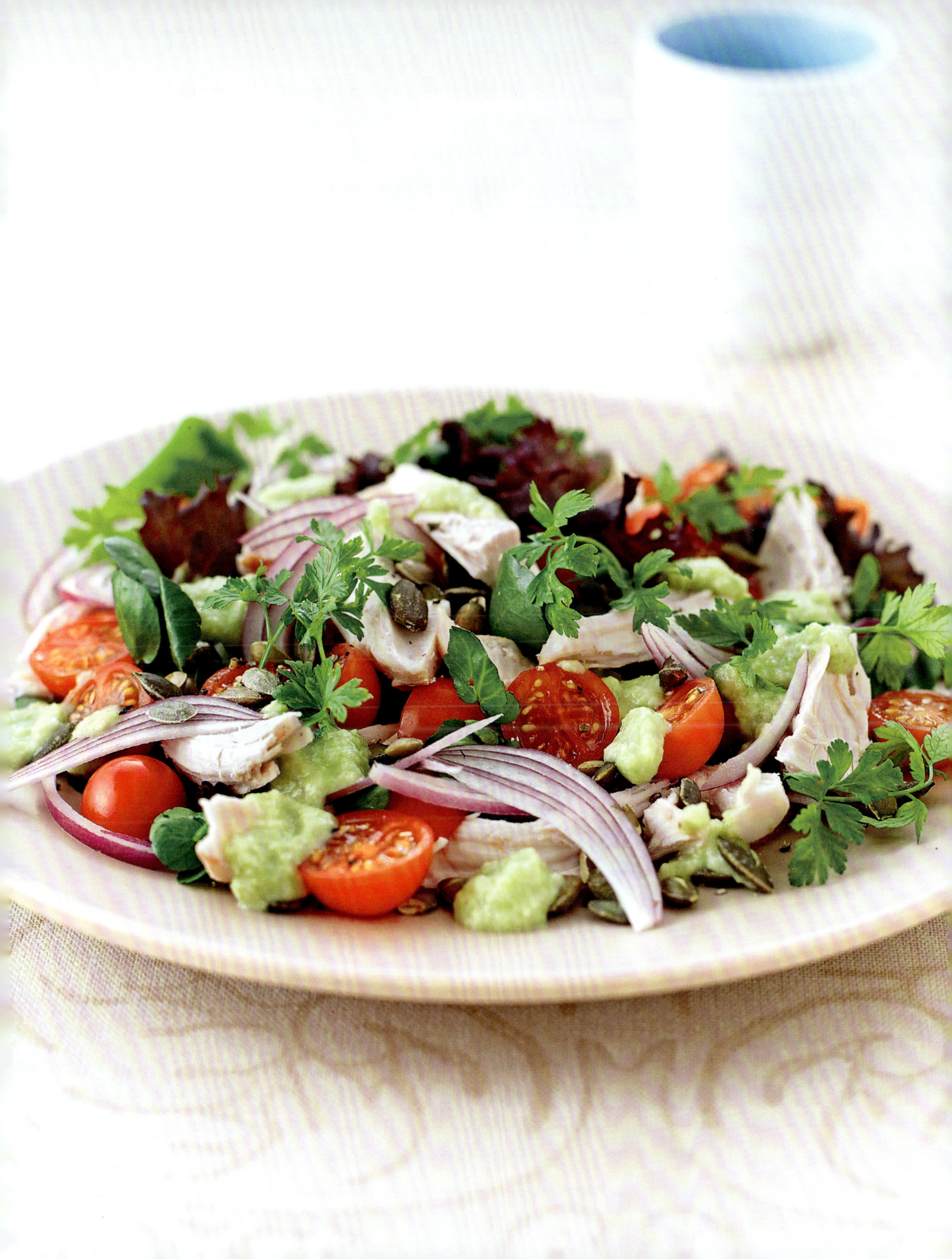

Makes 4 ▪ Preparation time: 15 minutes ▪ Cooking time: 7–8 minutes
Total time: 22–23 minutes

Goats' Cheese Flatbread Pizza

Ingredients

- **6 plum tomatoes**
- **small handful of fresh basil leaves**
- **1 garlic clove**
- **4 tablespoons olive oil**
- **4 × 20 cm (8 inch) Mediterranean flatbreads**
- **2 tablespoons sun-dried tomato paste**
- **300 g (10 oz) mozzarella cheese**
- **100 g (3½ oz) soft goats' cheese**
- **salt and pepper**

Equipment

- **kitchen scales**
- **1 chopping board**
- **1 sharp knife**
- **1 mixing bowl**
- **1 mixing spoon**
- **measuring spoons**
- **1 spoon**
- **2 baking sheets**

1. **Clear** your counter of clutter and **set out** all the equipment you need.
2. **Preheat** the oven to **200°C (400°F), Gas Mark 6**.
3. **Roughly chop** the plum tomatoes and **tear** the basil leaves. **Crush** (using the flat side of the knife) and **finely chop** the garlic.
4. **Put** the tomatoes in a mixing bowl, **add** the basil, garlic and oil, **season** generously with salt and pepper and **mix**.
5. **Lay** the flatbreads on 2 baking sheets and **spread** with the sun-dried tomato paste. **Slice** the mozzarella and **arrange** on top of the flatbreads. **Bake** in the oven for 7–8 minutes, until the bases are crisp and the cheese has melted.
6. **Divide** the tomato mixture between the flatbreads and **crumble** over the goats' cheese. **Serve** immediately.

Serves 4 ▪ Preparation time: 15 minutes ▪ Cooking time: 9 minutes
Total time: 24 minutes

Sardine Pitta Breads

Ingredients

- **2 boneless sardine fillets, about 100 g (3½ oz) each**
- **1 teaspoon ground cumin**
- **pinch of cayenne**
- **pinch of plain flour**
- **3 tablespoons olive oil**
- **10 g (¼ oz) preserved lemon**
- **handful of fresh coriander**
- **handful of fresh flat leaf parsley**
- **4 pitta breads**
- **1 tomato**
- **¼ cucumber**
- **salt and pepper**

Equipment

- **kitchen scales**
- **kitchen paper**
- **2 small bowls**
- **measuring spoons**
- **2 mixing spoons**
- **1 large nonstick frying pan**
- **1 spatula**
- **1 chopping board**
- **1 sharp knife**

TIP: Swap the sardines out for canned tuna or mackerel to mix this recipe up (and omit the cooking).

1. **Clear** your counter of clutter and **set out** all the equipment you need.
2. **Pat** the sardines dry with kitchen paper and **season** with salt and pepper. **Mix** together the cumin, cayenne and flour in a small bowl. **Dust** the fish all over with the spice mixture.
3. **Heat** 1 tablespoon of the oil in a large nonstick frying pan. **Cook** the sardine fillets, skin-side down, for 5 minutes. **Turn** the fish over and **cook** for a further 3 minutes until cooked through. **Remove** from the heat, **cover** with the lid and **keep warm**.
4. **Finely chop** the preserved lemon. **Chop** the coriander and parsley. **Mix** with the remaining oil in another small bowl and **season** well with salt and pepper.
5. **Lightly toast** the pitta breads and **split** them open.
6. **Chop** the tomato and **slice** the cucumber.
7. **Fill** the pitta breads with the sardines, tomato and cucumber, then **drizzle** over the lemon-herb dressing to **serve**.

Serves 4 • Preparation time: 10 minutes • Cooking time: 25 minutes
Total time: 35 minutes

Tomato & Basil Soup

Ingredients

- **500 ml (17 fl oz) hot vegetable or chicken stock**
- **1 large onion**
- **2 garlic cloves**
- **400 g (13 oz) can chickpeas**
- **2 tablespoons olive or vegetable oil**
- **500 g (1 lb) jar or carton passata or sieved Italian tomatoes**
- **small bunch of fresh basil**
- **salt and pepper**

Equipment

- **1 measuring jug**
- **1 chopping board**
- **1 sharp knife**
- **can opener**
- **1 sieve**
- **1 large saucepan**
- **measuring spoons**
- **1 wooden spoon**
- **timer**
- **1 hand-held stick blender**

TIP: Batch cook this in advance and have as a warming lunch with cheese on toast.

1. **Clear** your counter of clutter and **set out** all the equipment you need.
2. **Prepare** the stock according to the packet instructions.
3. **Chop** the onion and garlic.
4. **Drain** and **rinse** the chickpeas.
5. **Heat** the oil in a large saucepan and **cook** the onion over a **medium heat** for 7–8 minutes until softened. **Add** the garlic and **cook** gently for a further 2 minutes until softened.
6. **Pour** the passata or sieved Italian tomatoes and chickpeas into the pan with the hot stock, then bring to the **boil** and **simmer** gently for 15 minutes until rich and thickened slightly. **Set a timer** to every 5 minutes to remind you to give it a **stir**.
7. **Roughly chop** the basil leaves and **add** to the soup, reserving a little to garnish. **Season** to taste with salt and pepper, then **blend** with a hand-held stick blender until smooth and thick, adding a little extra hot water for the desired consistency, if needed. (Don't worry if you do not have a blender; this soup can be served as a chunky version.)
8. **Garnish** with the reserved chopped basil leaves, then **serve**.

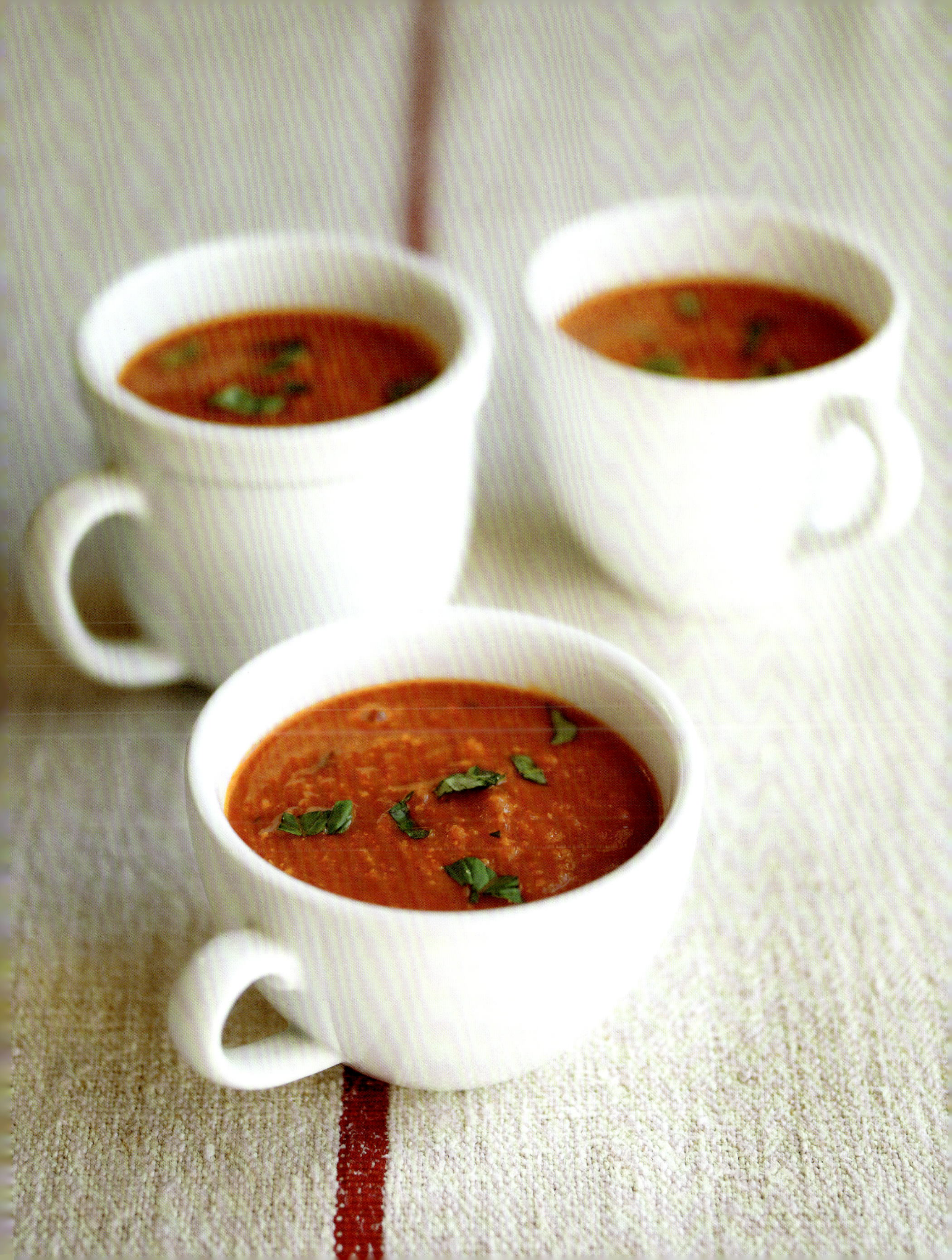

Serves 4 ▪ Preparation time: 15 minutes ▪ Cooking time: None
Total time: 15 minutes

Chicken Caesar Salad

Ingredients

- **2 anchovy fillets in oil**
- **40 g (1½ oz) Parmesan cheese, plus extra to serve**
- **½ lemon**
- **6 tablespoons low-fat crème fraîche**
- **2 Romaine lettuces**
- **1 ripe avocado**
- **375 g (12 oz) ready-cooked chargrilled chicken slices**
- **50 g (2 oz) ready-made baked croûtons**
- **pepper**

Equipment

- **kitchen scales**
- **1 grater**
- **1 lemon juicer**
- **1 food processor**
- **measuring spoons**
- **1 chopping board**
- **1 sharp knife**
- **1 mixing bowl**
- **salad servers**

1. **Clear** your counter of clutter and **set out** all the equipment you need.
2. Begin by making the dressing. **Drain** the anchovy fillets. **Grate** the Parmesan and lemon rind, then **juice** the lemon. **Place** the crème fraîche in a food processor with the drained anchovy fillets, grated Parmesan and lemon juice. **Blend** to make a smooth dressing and **season** to taste with pepper.
3. **Tear** the lettuce into bite-sized pieces and **peel**, **stone** and **chop** the avocado.
4. **Place** the lettuce in a mixing bowl with the avocado. **Pour** over the dressing, **toss** together and divide between 4 serving bowls.
5. **Arrange** the chicken on top and **scatter** with the croûtons. **Season** with pepper and **grate** over a little extra Parmesan. **Serve** immediately.

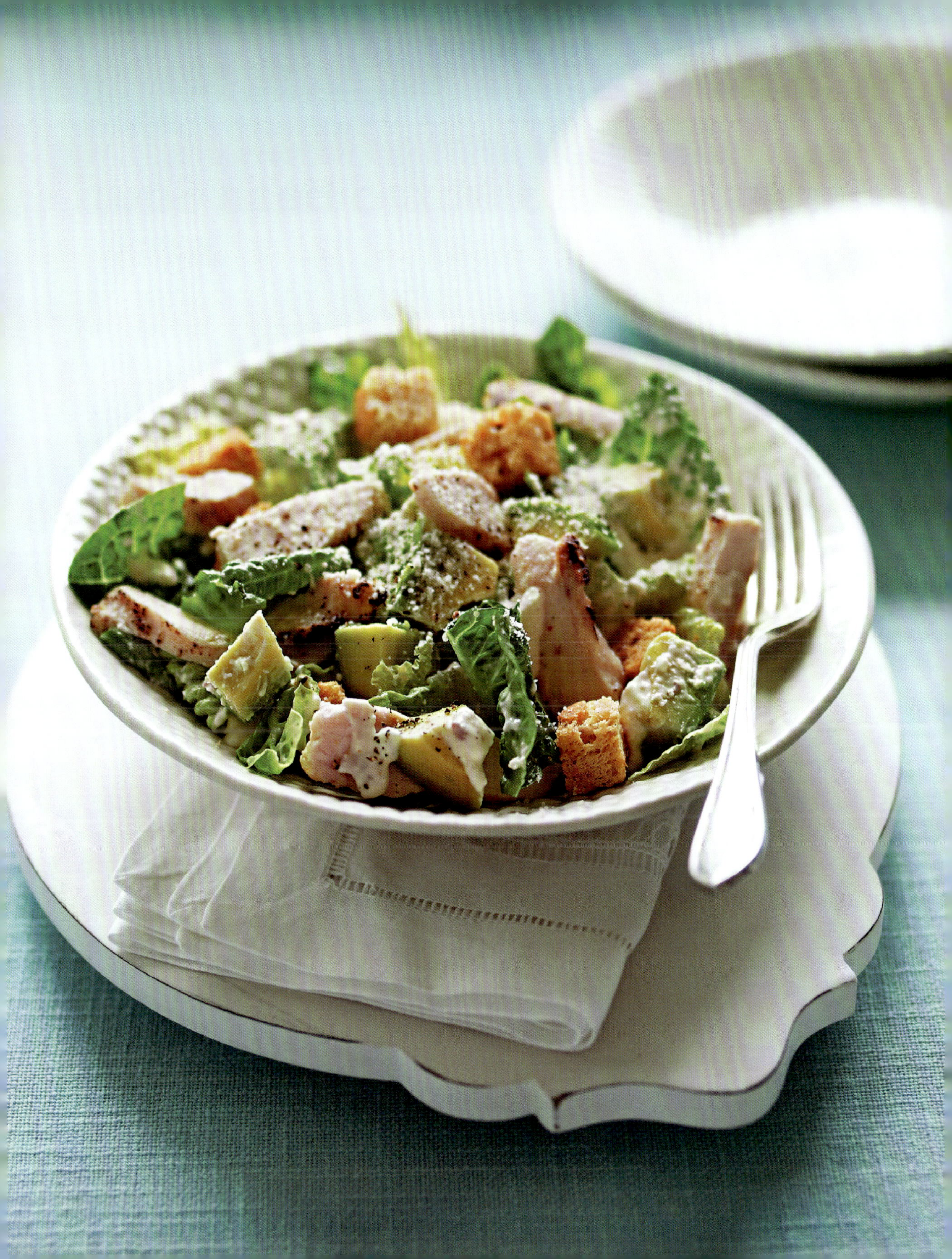

Serves 6 ▪ Preparation time: 15 minutes ▪ Cooking time: 40 minutes
Total time: 55 minutes

Squash, Kale & Mixed Bean Soup

Ingredients

- **900 ml (1½ pints) hot vegetable or chicken stock**
- **1 onion**
- **2 garlic cloves**
- **500 g (1 lb) butternut squash**
- **2 small carrots**
- **400 g (13oz) can mixed beans**
- **1 tablespoon olive oil**
- **1 teaspoon smoked paprika**
- **500 g (1 lb) canned chopped tomatoes**
- **100 g (3½ oz) kale**
- **150 ml (¼ pint) full-fat crème fraîche**
- **salt and pepper**

Equipment

- **kitchen scales**
- **measuring jugs**
- **1 chopping board**
- **1 sharp knife**
- **1 vegetable peeler**
- **can opener**
- **1 colander**
- **1 large saucepan with a lid**
- **1 wooden spoon**
- **measuring spoons**
- **timer**

TIPS: Many high-street supermarkets sell pre-diced fresh or frozen butternut squash to save time. Serve with warm garlic bread, cooked according to the packet instructions.

1. **Clear** your counter of clutter and **set out** all the equipment you need.
2. **Prepare** the stock according to the packet instructions.
3. **Finely chop** the onion and garlic. **Slice**, **deseed**, **peel** and **dice** the squash. **Dice** the carrots.
4. **Drain** and **rinse** the mixed beans in a colander.
5. **Heat** the oil in a large saucepan, **add** the onion and **fry** gently for 5 minutes. **Stir** in the garlic and smoked paprika and **cook** briefly, then **add** the squash, carrots, tomatoes and drained beans.
6. **Pour** in the stock, **season** with salt and pepper and bring to the **boil**, **stirring**. **Cover** and **simmer** for 25 minutes until the vegetables are tender. **Set a timer** every 5–10 minutes to remind you to give it a **stir**.
7. **Tear** the kale into bite-sized pieces.
8. **Stir** the crème fraîche into the soup, then **add** the kale, **pressing** it just beneath the surface of the stock. **Cover** and **cook** for 5 minutes until the kale has just wilted.
9. **Serve** with warm garlic bread, if liked.

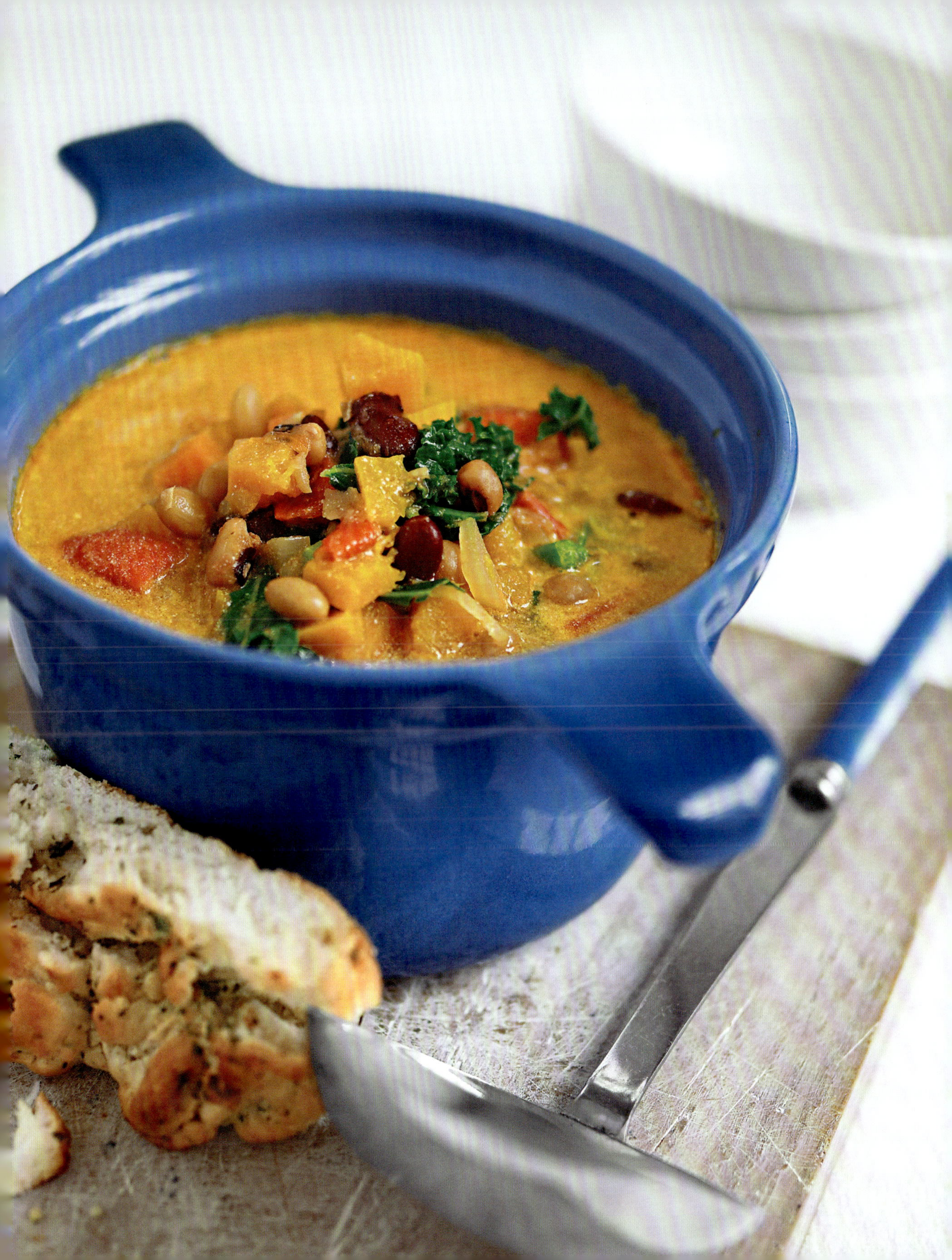

Serves 4 ▪ Preparation time: 10–15 minutes ▪ Cooking time: None
Total time: 10–15 minutes

Sardine & Three Bean Salad

Ingredients

- 1 red onion
- 2 celery sticks (optional)
- 400 g (13 oz) can butter beans or cannellini beans
- 200 g (7 oz) canned kidney beans or black beans
- 300 g (10 oz) canned beans (such as broad beans or chickpeas)
- 2 × 120 g (3¾ oz) cans sardines in oil or brine
- 1 tablespoon red wine vinegar
- 3 tablespoons olive oil
- salt and pepper
- 4 flatbreads, to serve (optional)

Equipment

- 1 chopping board
- 1 sharp knife
- can opener
- 1 colander
- 1 large bowl
- measuring spoons
- 1 mixing spoon

1. **Clear** your counter of clutter and **set out** all the equipment you need.
2. **Finely chop** the red onion and **finely slice** the celery, if using.
3. **Drain** and **rinse** all the beans in a colander. **Drain** and **flake** the sardines.
4. Gently **mix** all of the ingredients together in a large bowl and then **season** to taste with salt and pepper.
5. **Spoon** into bowls and **serve** with the flatbreads, if liked.

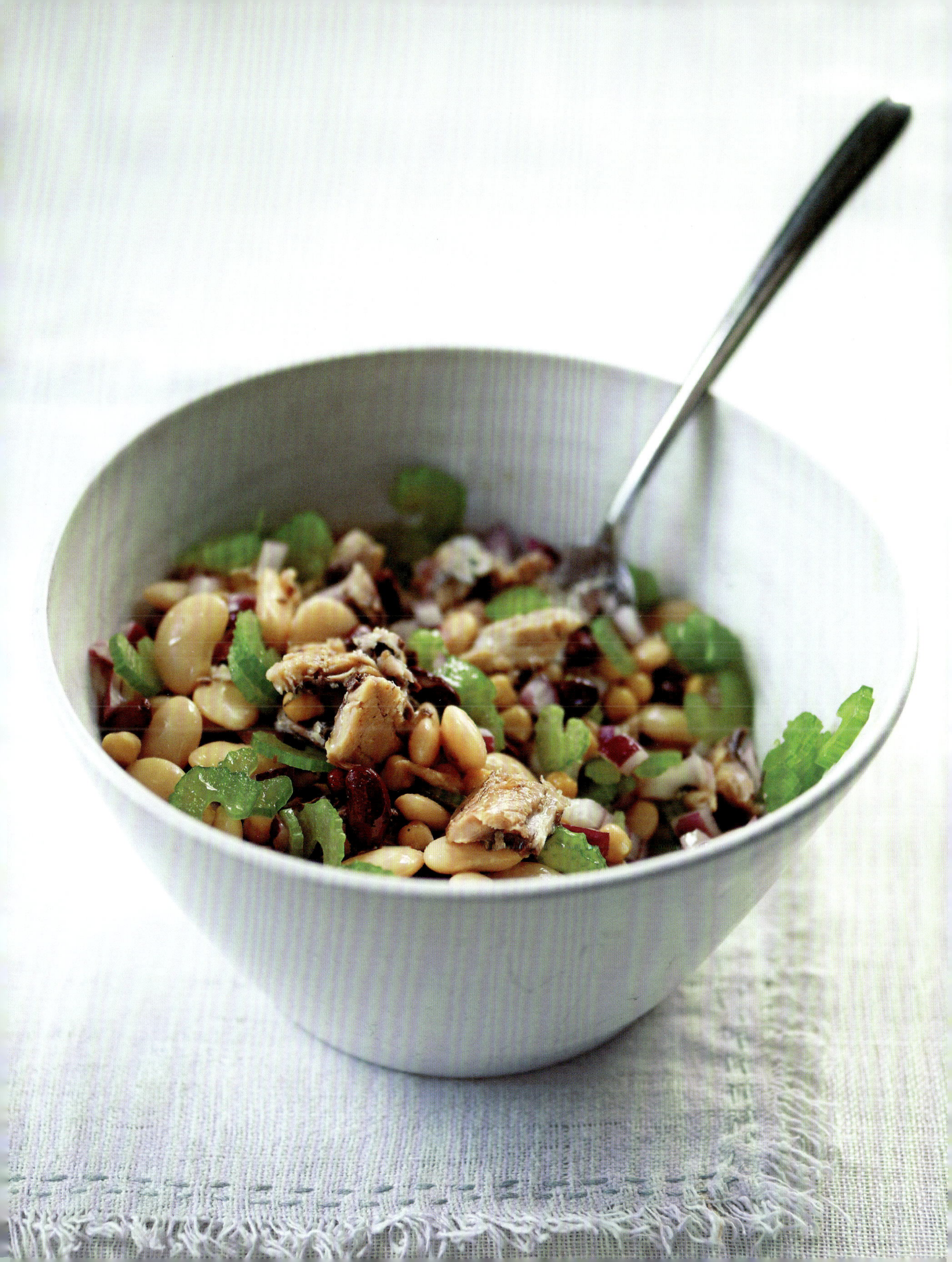

Serves 4 ▪ Preparation time: 10 minutes ▪ Cooking time: 5 minutes
Total time: 15 minutes

Salmon Pasta Salad with Dill Dressing

Ingredients

- **handful of fresh dill**
- **75 g (3 oz) crème fraîche**
- **4 tablespoons mayonnaise**
- **350 g (11½ oz) fresh fusilli**
- **2 spring onions**
- **¼ cucumber**
- **150 g (5 oz) smoked salmon**
- **salt and pepper**

Equipment

- **kitchen scales**
- **2 chopping boards**
- **2 sharp knives**
- **1 bowl**
- **measuring spoons**
- **1 mixing spoon**
- **1 large saucepan**
- **1 colander**
- **1 serving dish**

1. **Clear** your counter of clutter and **set out** all the equipment you need.
2. Begin by making the dressing. **Finely chop** the dill and **add** to a bowl. **Add** the crème fraîche and mayonnaise, **mix** together and **season** with salt and pepper. **Set aside**.
3. **Cook** the pasta in a large saucepan of salted boiling water according to the packet instructions until al dente.
4. **Slice** the spring onions and the cucumber. **On a separate chopping board, with a new knife**, **cut** the smoked salmon into strips.
5. **Drain** the pasta in a colander, then **cool** under cold running water and **drain** again.
6. **Tip** the pasta into a serving dish and **stir** through the spring onions, cucumber, smoked salmon and dill dressing, then **serve**.

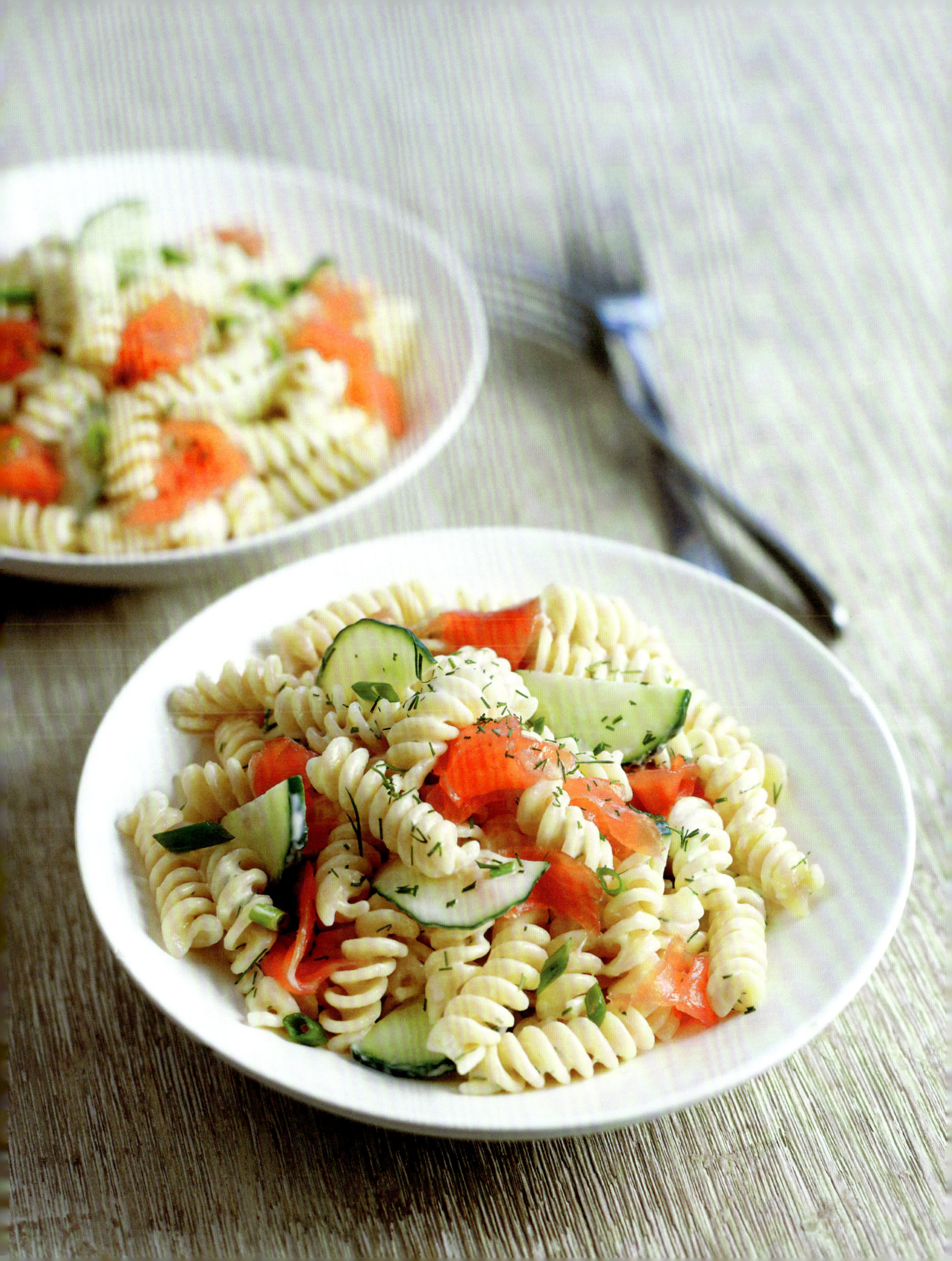

Serves 2 ▪ Preparation time: 10 minutes ▪ Cooking time: 5–7 minutes
Total time: 15–17 minutes

Refried Bean Quesadillas

Ingredients

- **2 spring onions**
- **10 g (¼ oz) fresh coriander**
- **50 g (2 oz) canned sweetcorn**
- **200 g (7 oz) can refried beans**
- **2 soft corn tortillas**
- **3 tablespoons ready-made fresh tomato salsa, plus extra to serve**
- **50 g (2 oz) Cheddar or Monterey Jack cheese**
- **olive oil, for brushing**

Equipment

- **kitchen scales**
- **1 chopping board**
- **1 sharp knife**
- **can opener**
- **1 sieve**
- **1 mixing bowl**
- **1 mixing spoon**
- **measuring spoons**
- **1 grater**
- **1 large frying pan**
- **1 pastry brush**
- **1 spatula**

1. **Clear** your counter of clutter and **set out** all the equipment you need.
2. **Chop** the spring onions and coriander. **Drain** the canned sweetcorn in a sieve. **Add** these vegetables to a mixing bowl with the refried beans and **mix** together.
3. **Place** 1 corn tortilla flat on the counter and **cover** it with the bean mixture, then **top** with the tomato salsa and **grate** over the cheese. **Cover** with the remaining corn tortilla to make a quesadilla.
4. **Brush** a large frying pan with oil and **heat** over a **medium heat**. When hot, **add** the quesadilla and **cook** for 2–3 minutes, **pressing** down with a spatula, until the cheese starts to melt.
5. **Flip** the quesadilla in the pan and **cook** it on the other side for 2–3 minutes.
6. **Remove** the quesadilla from the pan and **cut** it into wedges. **Serve** with extra tomato salsa.

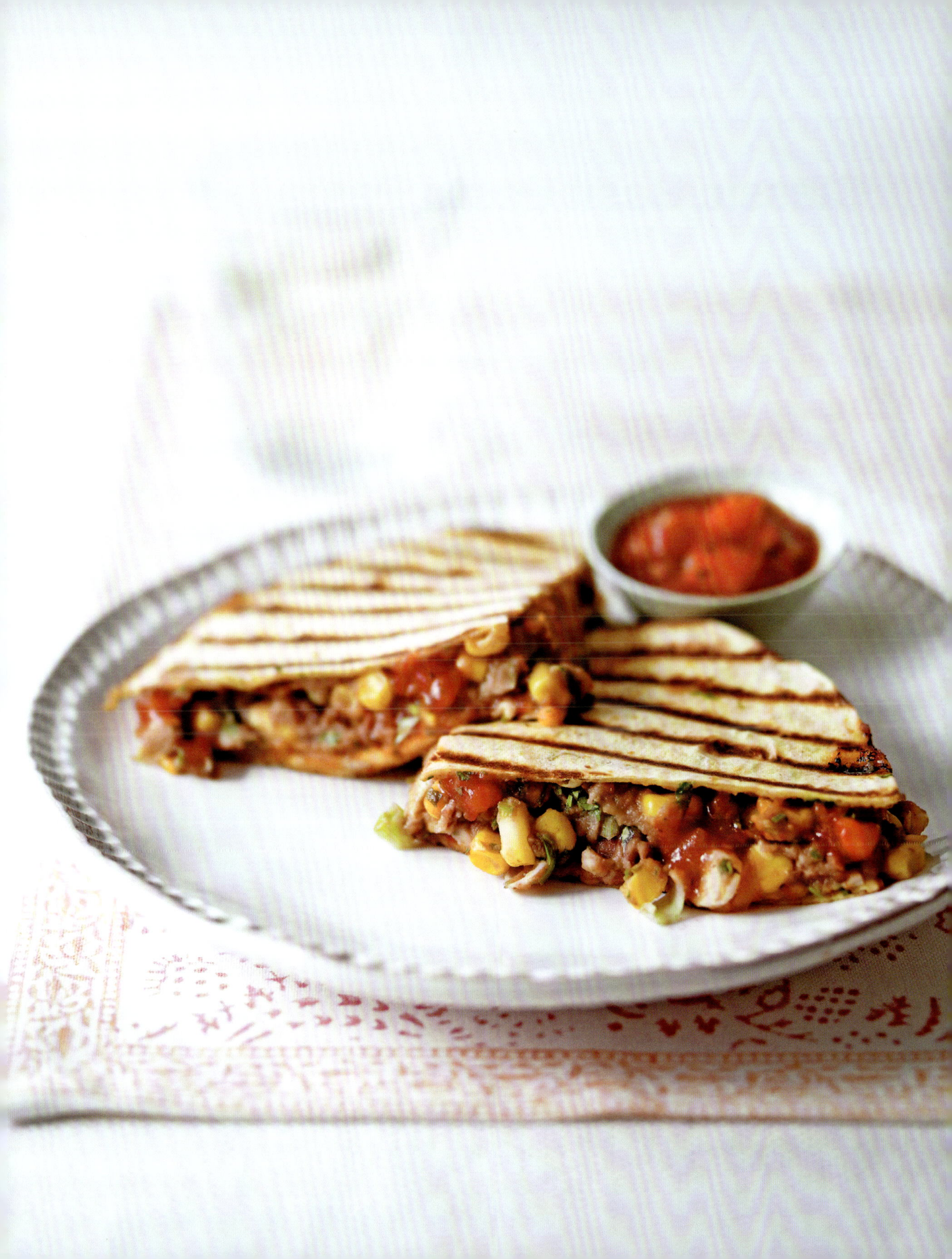

Serves 4 ▪ Preparation time: 10 minutes ▪ Cooking time: 10–12 minutes
Total time: 20–22 minutes

Classic Basil Pesto Pasta

Ingredients

- **75 g (3 oz) fresh basil leaves, plus extra to garnish**
- **50 g (2 oz) pine nuts**
- **2 garlic cloves**
- **50 g (2 oz) Parmesan cheese, plus extra to serve**
- **100 ml (3½ fl oz) olive oil**
- **400 g (13 oz) dried trofie**
- **salt and pepper**

Equipment

- **kitchen scales**
- **1 measuring jug**
- **1 food processor**
- **1 rubber spatula**
- **1 grater**
- **1 large saucepan**
- **1 ladle**

TIP: This makes a great base recipe to add your favourite protein to, such as pre-cooked chicken, tofu or salmon flakes. Try different variations to avoid getting bored.

1. **Clear** your counter of clutter and **set out** all the equipment you need.
2. **Put** the basil, pine nuts and garlic in a food processor and **blend** until well combined. **Transfer** to a bowl using a rubber spatula, **grate** in the Parmesan and **stir** in the oil. **Season** with salt and pepper.
3. **Cook** the pasta in a large saucepan of salted boiling water according to the packet instructions until al dente.
4. **Reserving** a ladleful of the cooking water, **drain** the pasta, and **return** it to the pan. **Stir** in the pesto, adding enough of the reserved pasta cooking water to loosen the mixture.
5. **Serve** immediately, **scattered** with extra grated Parmesan and **garnished** with extra basil leaves.

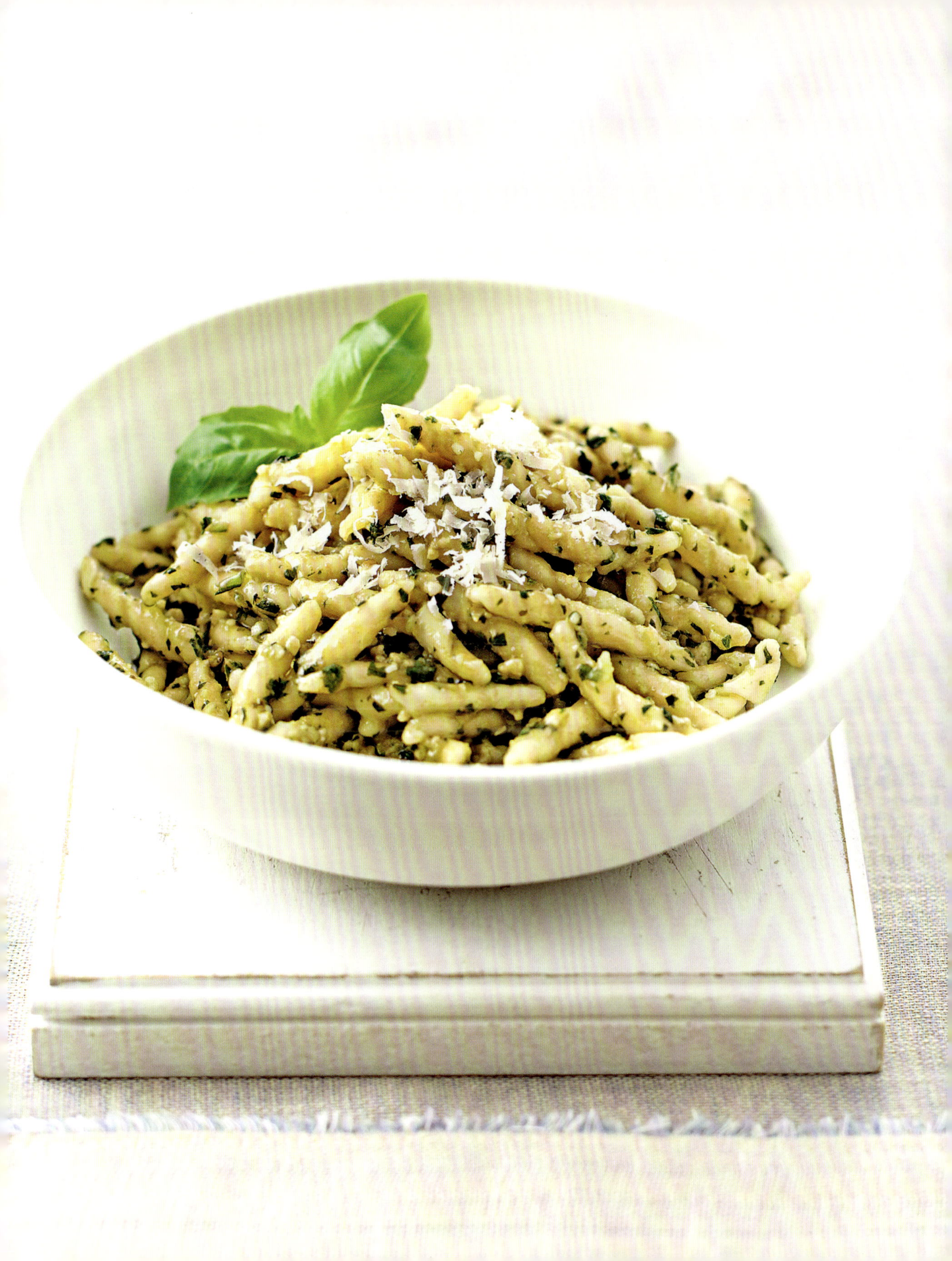

Serves 4 ▪ Preparation time: 15 minutes ▪ Cooking time: 15–18 minutes
Total time: 30–33 minutes

Hearty Minestrone

Ingredients

- **1.5 litres (2½ pints) hot vegetable stock**
- **3 carrots**
- **1 red onion**
- **6 celery sticks**
- **2 garlic cloves**
- **200 g (7 oz) potatoes**
- **2 tablespoons olive oil**
- **4 tablespoons tomato purée**
- **400 g (13 oz) can chopped tomatoes**
- **150 g (5 oz) dried soup pasta**
- **400 g (13 oz) can cannellini beans**
- **100 g (3½ oz) baby spinach**
- **salt and pepper**
- **crusty bread, to serve**

Equipment

- **kitchen scales**
- **1 measuring jug**
- **1 chopping board**
- **1 sharp knife**
- **1 food processor**
- **1 vegetable peeler**
- **1 large saucepan with a lid**
- **measuring spoons**
- **can opener**
- **1 wooden spoon**
- **timer**
- **1 colander**

1. **Clear** your counter of clutter and **set out** all the equipment you need.
2. **Prepare** the stock according to the packet instructions.
3. **Roughly chop** the carrots, red onion, celery, and garlic, then **whizz** in a food processor until finely chopped.
4. **Peel** and **cut** the potatoes into 1 cm (½ inch) dice.
5. **Heat** the oil in a large saucepan over a **medium heat**, **add** the chopped vegetables, potatoes, tomato purée, stock, tomatoes and pasta. Bring to the **boil**, **reduce the heat** and **simmer**, **covered**, for 12–15 minutes. **Set a timer** for every 5 minutes to remember give it a **stir**.
6. **Drain** and **rinse** the cannellini beans in a colander, then **tip** into the saucepan along with the spinach for the final 2 minutes of the cooking time.
7. **Season** to taste with salt and pepper and **serve** with crusty bread.

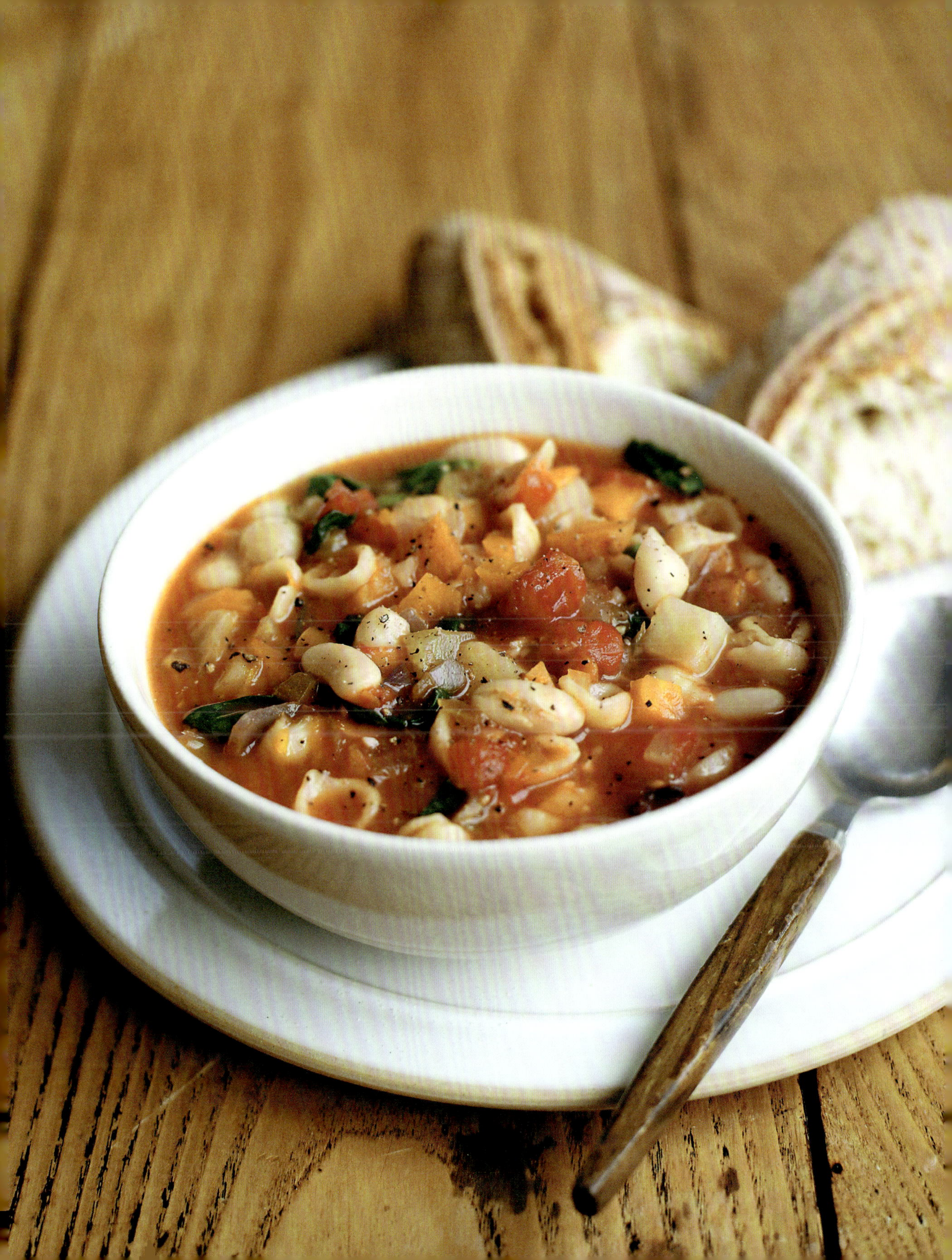

Serves 4 ▪ Preparation time: 10–15 minutes ▪ Cooking time: 5–6 minutes
Total time: 16–21 minutes

Warm Lentil, Tomato & Halloumi Salad

Ingredients

- **½ red onion**
- **250 g (8 oz) cherry tomatoes**
- **small handful of fresh coriander leaves**
- **small handful of fresh mint leaves**
- **1 garlic clove**
- **½ lemon**
- **400 g (13 oz) can green lentils**
- **2 tablespoons extra virgin olive oil**
- **250 g (8 oz) halloumi cheese**

Equipment

- **kitchen scales**
- **1 chopping board**
- **1 sharp knife**
- **1 lemon juicer**
- **can opener**
- **1 sieve**
- **measuring spoons**
- **1 mixing bowl**
- **1 mixing spoon**
- **1 nonstick frying pan**
- **1 silicone spatula**

1. **Clear** your counter of clutter and **set out** all the equipment you need.
2. **Slice** the red onion and **halve** the cherry tomatoes. **Roughly chop** the coriander and mint leaves.
3. **Crush** (using the flat side of the knife) and **finely chop** the garlic. **Juice** the lemon. **Drain** and **rinse** the lentils.
4. **Toss** all the ingredients, except the halloumi, together in a mixing bowl.
5. **Cut** the halloumi into chunks.
6. **Heat** a nonstick frying pan over a **medium heat** and **dry-fry** the halloumi for 4–5 minutes, **turning** frequently, until golden.
7. **Stir** the cooked halloumi into the salad and **serve** immediately.

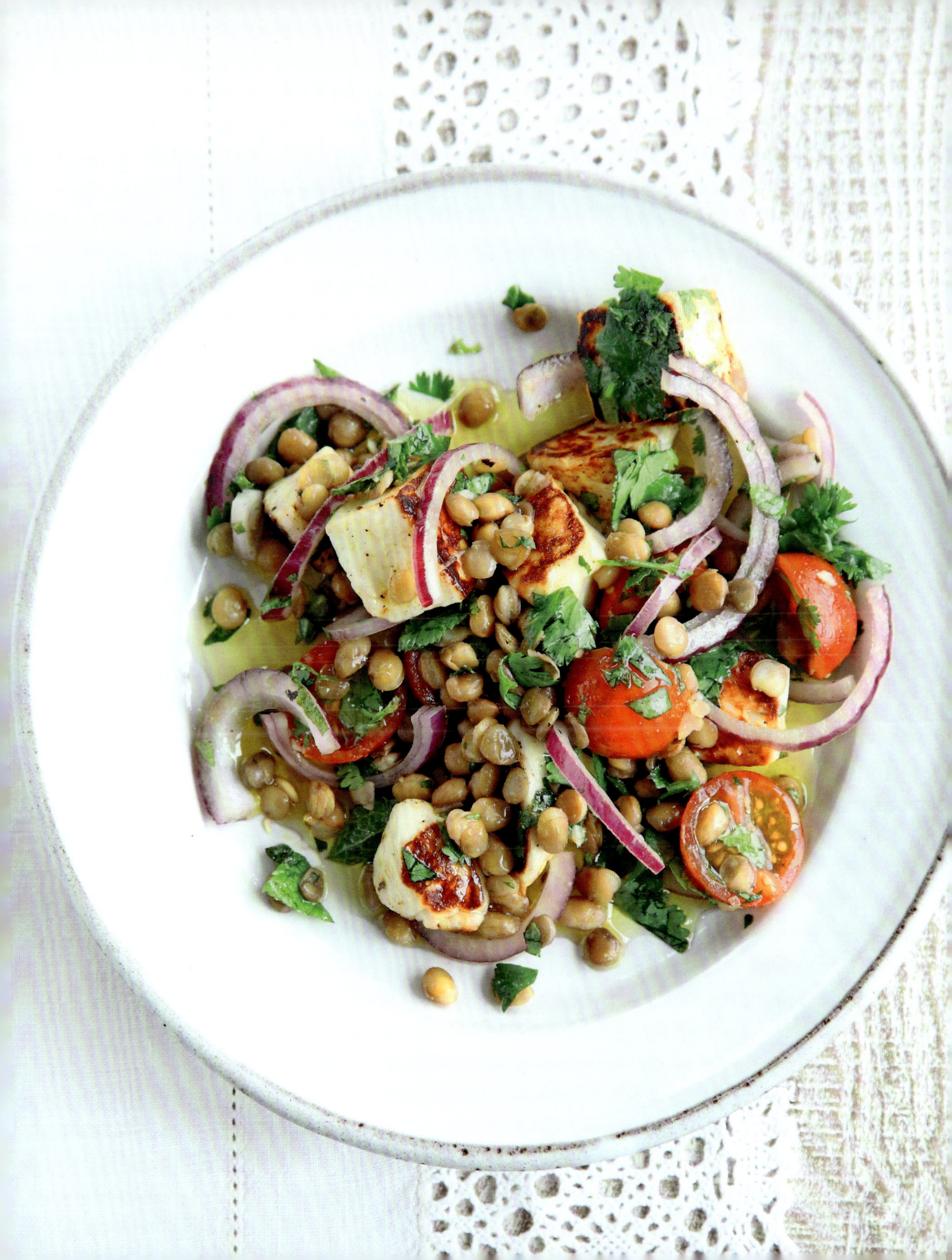

Serves 4 ▪ Preparation time: 10 minutes ▪ Cooking time: 10 minutes
Total time: 20 minutes

Vegetable & Tofu Stir-fry

Ingredients

- **300 g (10 oz) firm tofu**
- **1 onion**
- **3 tablespoons sunflower oil**
- **600 g (1 lb 5 oz) stir-fry vegetable mix**
- **2 tablespoons soy sauce**
- **2 tablespoons sweet chilli sauce**
- **125 ml (4 fl oz) water**
- **microwave rice, to serve**
- **1–2 red chillies, to garnish**
- **Thai or Italian fresh basil leaves, to garnish**

Equipment

- **kitchen scales**
- **1 measuring jug**
- **1 chopping board**
- **1 sharp knife**
- **1 wok or large frying pan**
- **meauring spoons**
- **1 wooden spoon**
- **1 slotted spoon**
- **1 small bowl**

1. **Clear** your counter of clutter and **set out** all the equipment you need.
2. **Drain** the tofu, **pat dry** with kitchen paper and **cut** into cubes. **Slice** the onion.
3. **Heat** 1 tablespoon of the oil in a wok or large frying pan until starting to smoke, **add** the tofu and **stir-fry** over a high heat for 2 minutes or until golden. **Remove** with a slotted spoon and **keep warm**.
4. **Heat** the remaining oil in the pan, **add** the onion and stir-fry veg mix and **stir-fry** according to the packet instructions.
5. **Mix** together the soy and chilli sauces and measured water in a small bowl and **add** to the pan with the stir-fried tofu. **Stir-fry** for 1 minute.
6. **Microwave** the rice according to the packet instructions. **Slice** the red chillies.
7. **Serve** the stir-fry in bowls with the rice, **garnished** with the red chillies and some basil leaves.

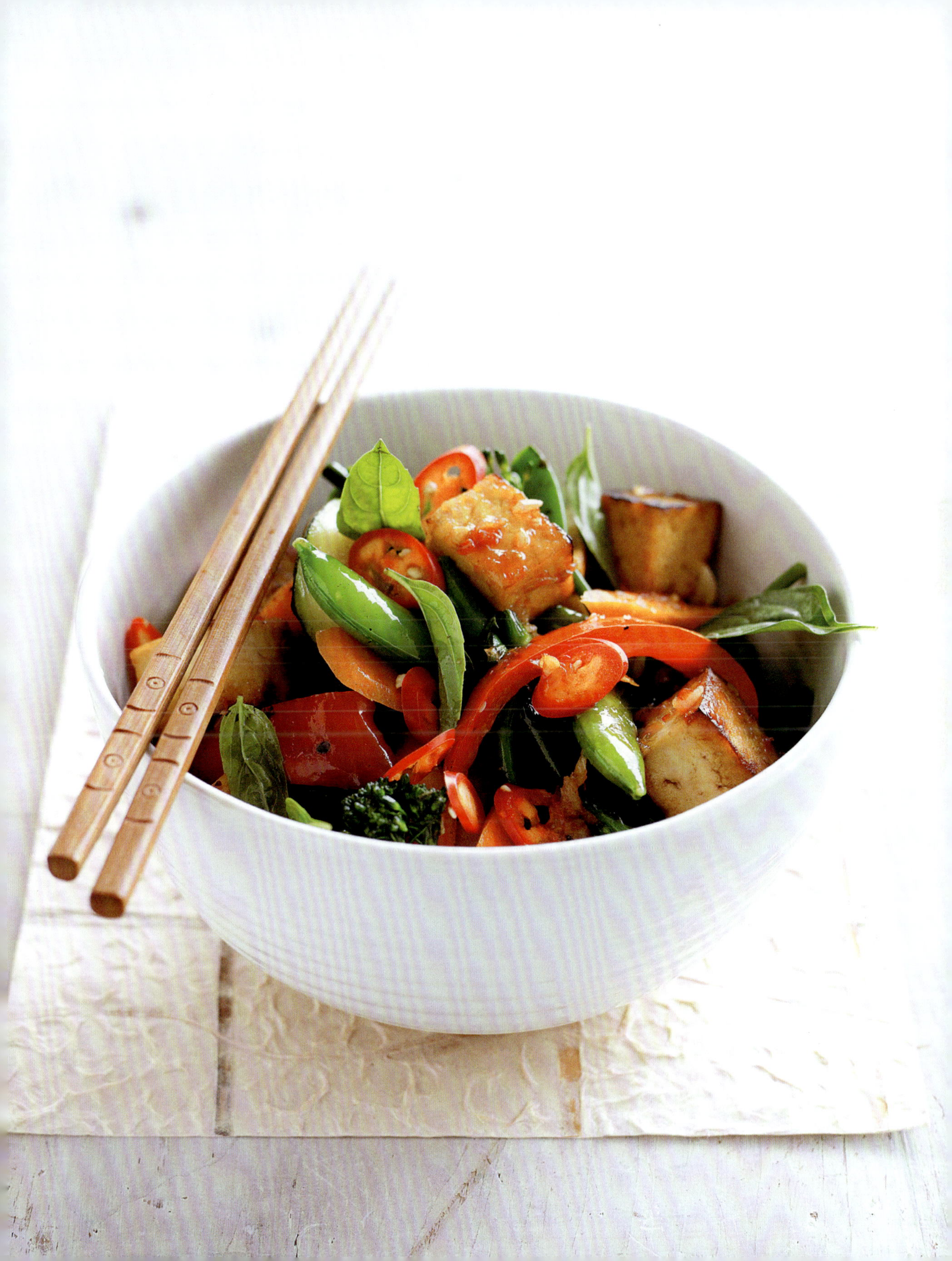

Serves 4 ▪ Preparation time: 10 minutes ▪ Cooking time: None
Total time: 10 minutes

Tuna & Cannellini Bean Salad

Ingredients

- **100 g (3½ oz) tomatoes**
- **1 red onion**
- **400 g (13 oz) can cannellini beans**
- **410 g (13¼ oz) can tuna**
- **30 g (1 oz) pitted black olives**
- **50 g (2 oz) rocket leaves**
- **extra virgin olive oil, for drizzling**
- **crusty bread, to serve (optional)**

Equipment

- **kitchen scales**
- **1 chopping board**
- **1 sharp knife**
- **can opener**
- **1 colander**
- **1 serving bowl**
- **1 fork**
- **1 mixing spoon**

1. **Clear** your counter of clutter and **set out** all the equipment you need.
2. **Chop** the tomatoes and **slice** the red onion.
3. **Drain** and **rinse** the cannellini beans in a colander.
4. **Drain** the tuna, **place** in a serving bowl and **break** it into chunks using a fork.
5. **Mix** in the chopped tomatoes, black olives, cannellini beans, red onion and rocket leaves.
6. **Drizzle** with extra virgin olive oil and **serve** immediately with crusty bread, if liked.

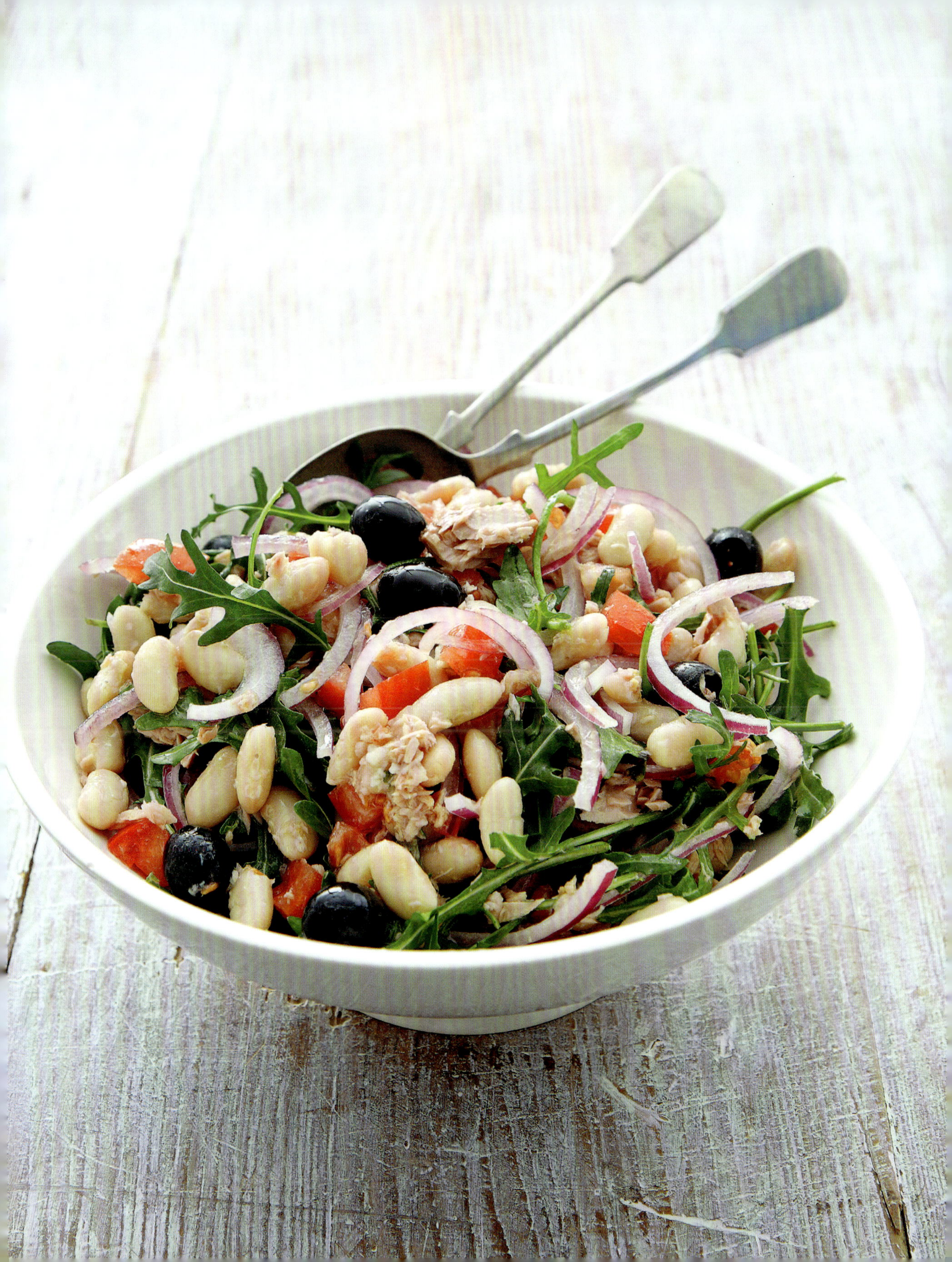

Serves 4 ▪ Preparation time: 10 minutes ▪ Cooking time: 25–30 minutes
Total time: 35–40 minutes

Chunky Spiced Bean Soup

Ingredients

- **750 ml (1¼ pints) hot vegetable stock**
- **1 large onion**
- **1 red pepper**
- **1 red chilli**
- **2 garlic cloves (optional)**
- **400 g (13 oz) can mixed beans**
- **2 tablespoons vegetable or olive oil**
- **500 g (1 lb) jar or carton passata or sieved Italian tomatoes**
- **200 g (7 oz) mixed chopped frozen or leftover vegetables**
- **salt and pepper**
- **fresh parsley, to serve (optional)**

Equipment

- **kitchen scales**
- **1 measuring jug**
- **1 chopping board**
- **1 sharp knife**
- **can opener**
- **1 colander**
- **1 large saucepan**
- **measuring spoons**
- **1 wooden spoon**
- **timer**

1. **Clear** your counter of clutter and **set out** all the equipment you need.
2. **Prepare** the stock according to the packet instructions.
3. **Chop** the onion, **core**, **deseed** and **chop** the red pepper and **deseed** and **chop** the chilli. **Chop** the garlic, if using.
4. **Drain** and **rinse** the mixed beans in a colander.
5. **Heat** the oil in a large saucepan and **add** the onion, pepper, chilli and garlic, if using. **Cook** gently over a **medium heat** for 6–7 minutes until softened.
6. **Stir** in the beans, passata or sieved Italian tomatoes and stock and bring to the **boil**. **Reduce** the heat slightly and **simmer** gently for 12–15 minutes until thickened slightly. **Set a timer** every 5–10 minutes to remind you to give it a **stir**.
7. **Add** the mixed chopped vegetables and **simmer** gently for a further 3–4 minutes until just tender. **Season** to taste with salt and pepper.
8. **Roughly chop** the parsley, if using, and sprinkle over the soup to **serve**.

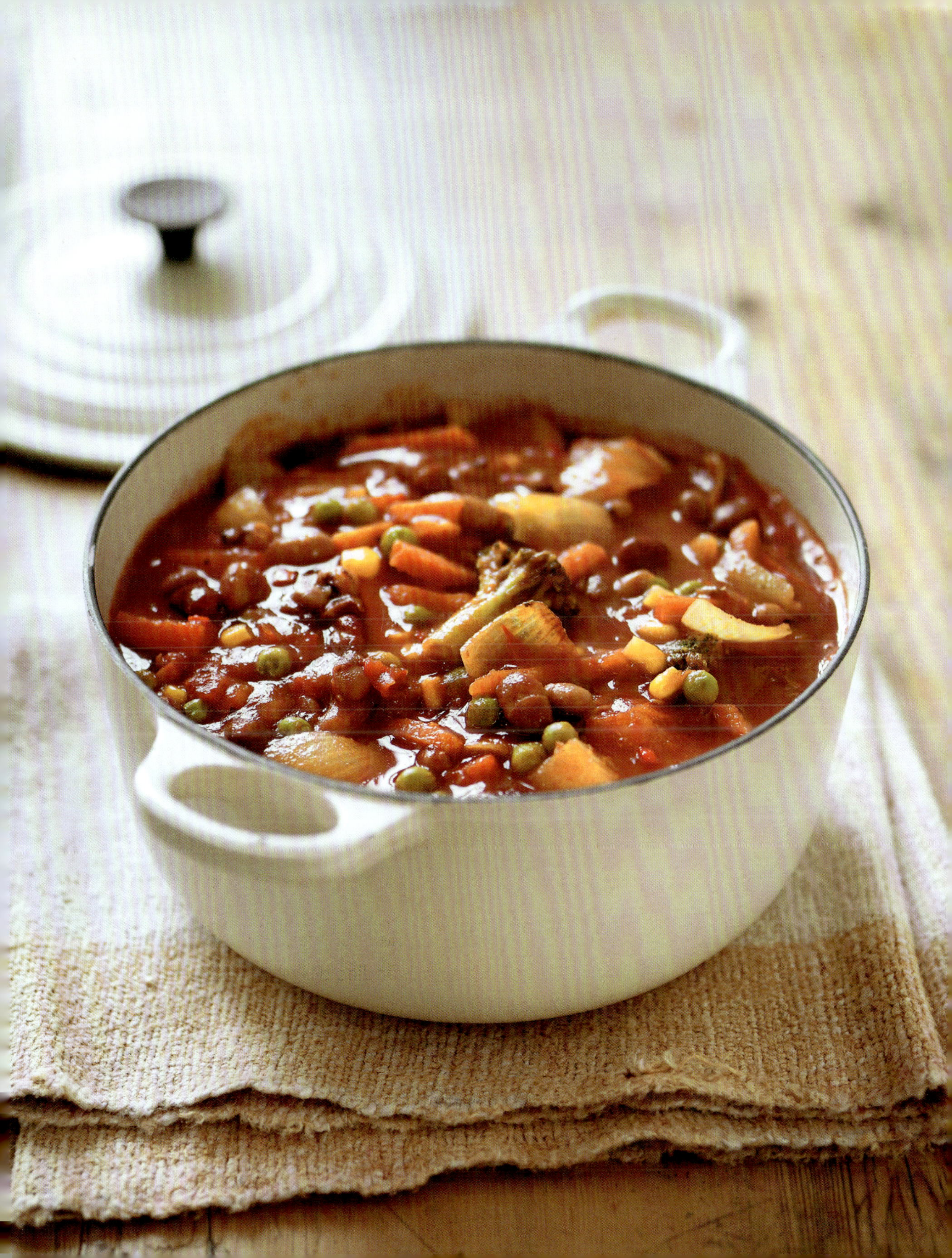

Serves 4 ▪ Preparation time: 10 minutes ▪ Cooking time: 12 minutes
Total time: 22 minutes

Sticky Lemon Chicken Noodles

Ingredients

- **300 g (10 oz) chicken fillets**
- **2 garlic cloves**
- **2.5cm (1 inch) piece of fresh root ginger**
- **1 red chilli**
- **1 lemon**
- **2 tablespoons vegetable oil**
- **200 g (7 oz) Tenderstem broccoli**
- **1 tablespoon clear honey**
- **2 teaspoons light soy sauce**
- **300 g (10 oz) ready-cooked egg noodles**
- **a splash of water**
- **handful of roasted cashew nuts**

Equipment

- **kitchen scales**
- **2 chopping boards**
- **2 sharp knives**
- **1 grater**
- **1 lemon juicer**
- **1 wok**
- **measuring spoons**
- **1 wooden spatula**

1. **Clear** your counter of clutter and **set out** all the equipment you need.
2. **Cut** the chicken fillets into thin strips.
3. **Using a separate chopping board and a new knife**, **crush** (using the flat side of the knife) and **finely chop** the garlic. **Peel** and **grate** the piece of fresh root ginger and **finely chop** the chilli. **Grate** the rind from the lemon and then **halve** and **juice** it.
4. **Heat** a wok until smoking hot, then **pour** in the oil, **swirl** it around the pan and **add** the chicken strips. **Cook** for 1 minute on a **high heat**, then **add** the broccoli and **cook** for 5 minutes until the chicken is nearly cooked through, **stirring** regularly.
5. **Add** the garlic, ginger and chilli to the wok and **cook** for a further 1 minute. Then **add** the lemon rind and juice, the honey and soy sauce and **toss** around the pan.
6. **Add** the noodles and the splash of water and **cook** until the noodles are heated through.
7. Divide the noodles between 4 serving bowls, scatter over the roasted cashew nuts and serve.

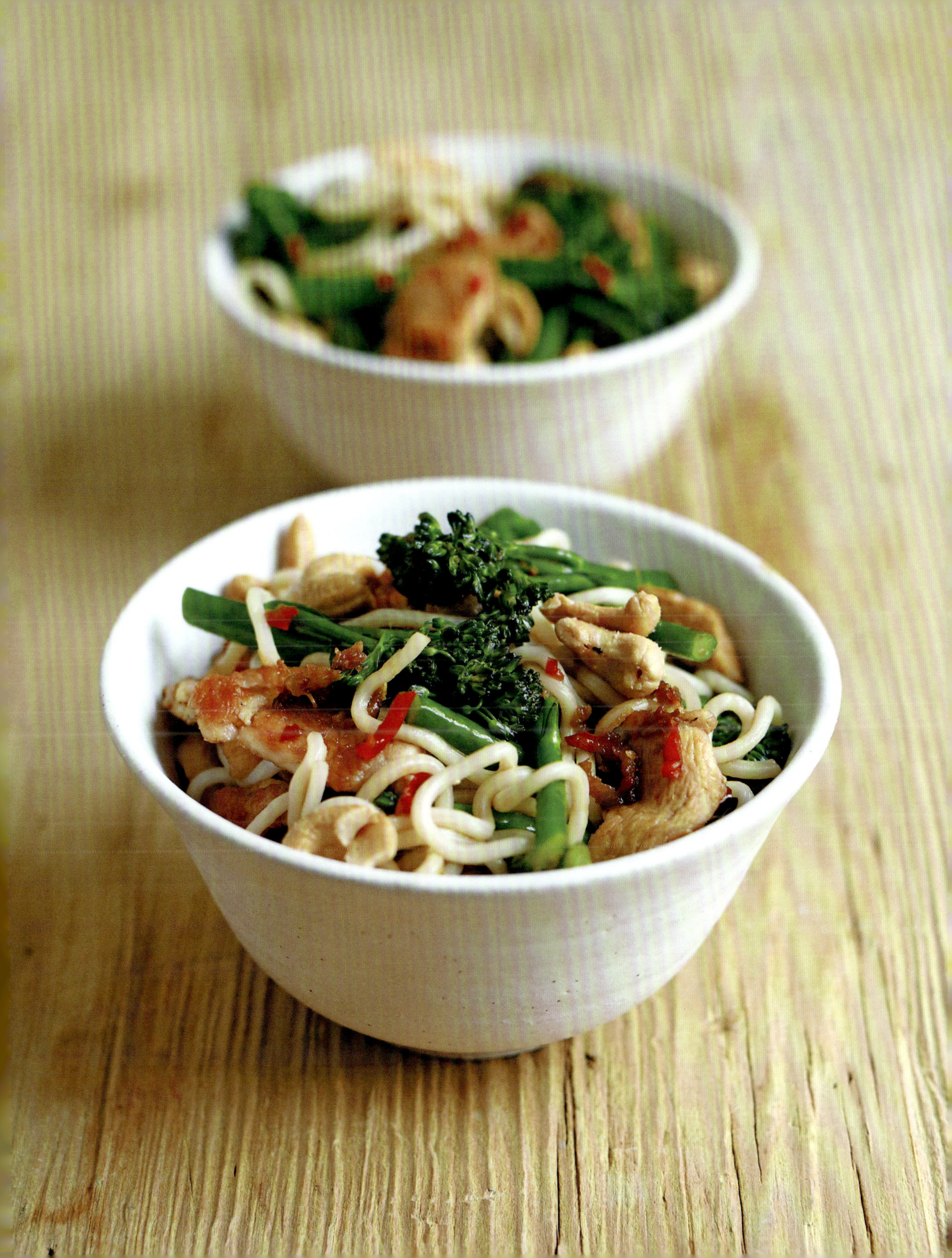

Serves 4 ▪ Preparation time: 10–15 minutes ▪ Cooking time: 25 minutes
Total time: 35–40 minutes

Chicken & Sweet Potato Curry

Ingredients

- 500 g (1 lb) boneless, skinless chicken breasts
- 1 large onion
- 1 medium red chilli
- 600 g (1 lb 5 oz) sweet potatoes
- 250 g (8 oz) green beans
- 2 tablespoons vegetable oil
- 2–4 tablespoons korma curry paste
- 400 ml (14 fl oz) can coconut milk
- 400 g (13 oz) can chopped tomatoes
- 20 g (¾ oz) fresh coriander leaves
- microwave rice, to serve

Equipment

- kitchen scales
- 2 chopping boards
- 2 sharp knives
- 1 vegetable peeler
- 1 large saucepan with a lid
- measuring spoons
- 2 wooden spoons

TIP: Many high-street supermarkets sell pre-diced sweet potato.

1. **Clear** your counter of clutter and **set out** all the equipment you need.
2. **Chop** the chicken breasts into chunks.
3. **Using a separate chopping board and a new knife, chop** the onion and **deseed** and **chop** the chilli. **Peel** the sweet potatoes and **cut** into chunks. **Trim** and **halve** the green beans.
4. **Heat** the oil in a large saucepan, **add** the onion and **cook** over a **medium heat** for 2–3 minutes until softened. **Add** the chilli, chicken and sweet potatoes and **cook** for 5 minutes, **stirring** occasionally.
5. **Add** the korma paste and **cook** for 1 minute, then **add** the coconut milk, tomatoes and green beans. Bring to the **boil**, then **reduce** the heat, **cover** and **simmer** for 15 minutes until the sweet potato is tender and the chicken is cooked through, **stirring** occasionally.
6. **Microwave** the rice according to the packet instructions.
7. **Chop** the coriander leaves, **stir** into the microwave rice and **serve** with the curry.

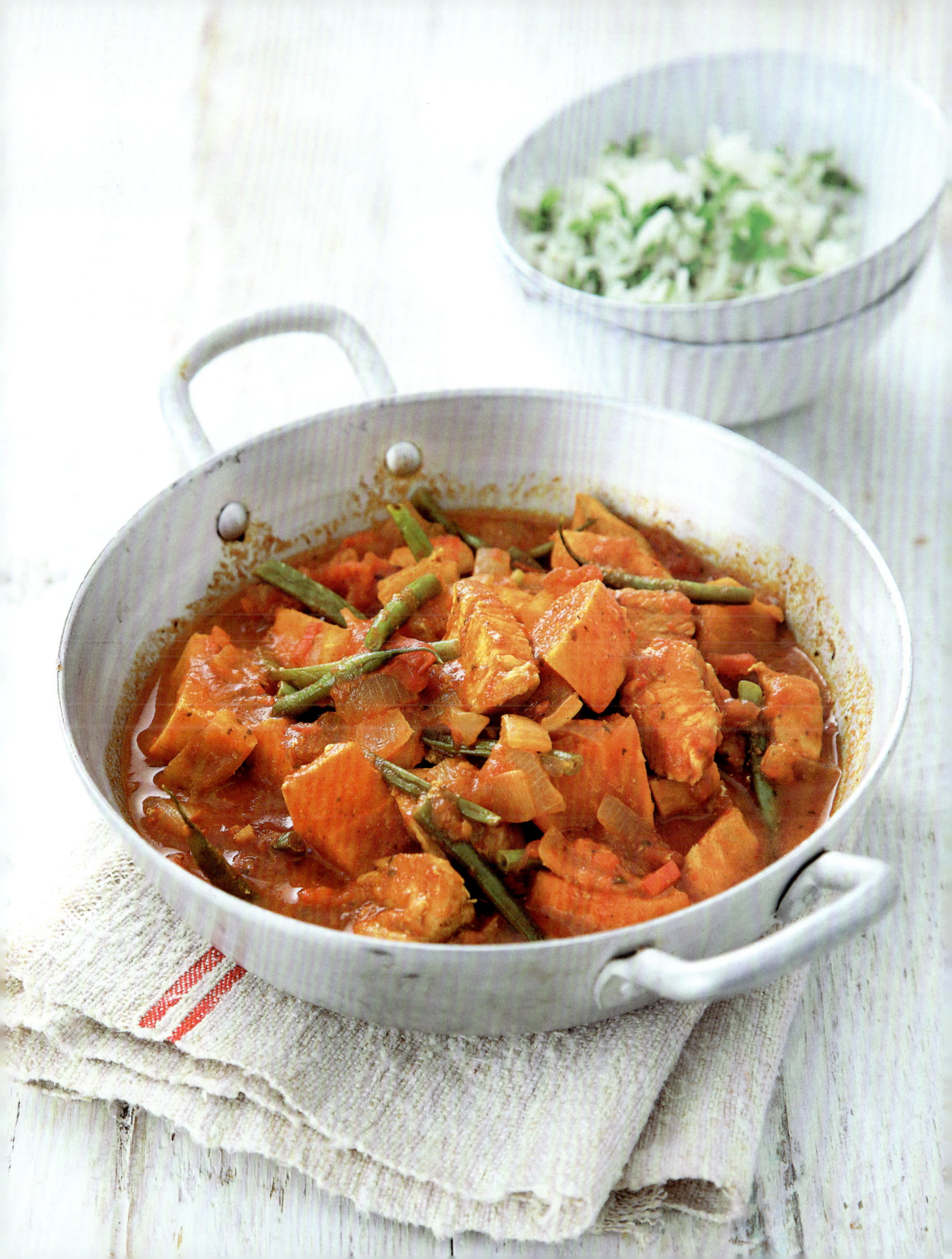

Dinner

Serves 4 ▪ Preparation time: 10 minutes ▪ Cooking time: 40 minutes
Total time: 50 minutes

Spiced Chickpeas with Kale

Ingredients

- **300 ml (½ pint) hot vegetable stock**
- **3 red onions**
- **400 g (13 oz) can chickpeas**
- **3 tablespoons vegetable oil**
- **2 tablespoons mild curry paste**
- **400 g (13 oz) can chopped tomatoes**
- **2 teaspoons soft light brown sugar**
- **100 g (3½ oz) curly kale**
- **salt and pepper**

Equipment

- **kitchen scales**
- **1 measuring jug**
- **1 chopping board**
- **1 sharp knife**
- **can opener**
- **1 colander**
- **1 large saucepan with a lid**
- **measuring spoons**
- **1 wooden spoon**
- **timer**

1. **Clear** your counter of clutter and **set out** all the equipment you need.
2. **Prepare** the stock according to the packet instructions.
3. **Cut** the red onions into wedges.
4. **Drain** and **rinse** the chickpeas in a colander.
5. **Heat** the oil in a large saucepan and **fry** the onions for 5 minutes over a **medium heat** until beginning to colour. **Stir** in the curry paste and then the tomatoes, chickpeas, stock and sugar.
6. Bring to the **boil**, then **reduce** the heat, **cover** and **simmer** gently for 20 minutes. **Set a timer** every 10 minutes to remember to stir.
7. **Slice** the kale, then **add** to the pan and **cook** gently for a further 10 minutes. **Season** to taste with salt and pepper and **serve**.

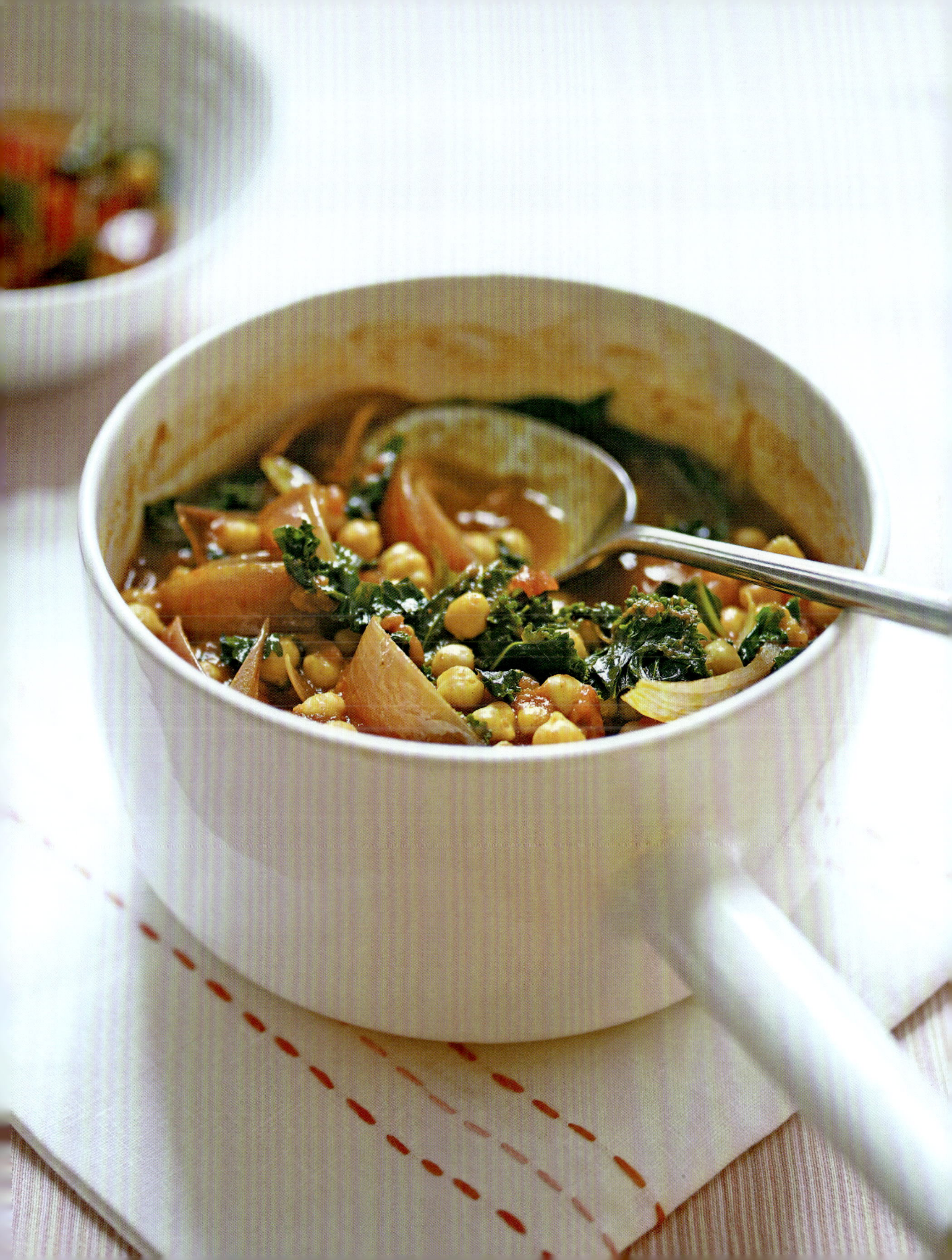

Serves 4 ▪ Preparation time: 10 minutes ▪ Cooking time: 5 minutes
Total time: 15 minutes

Seared Tuna with Lemon, Bean & Rocket Salad

Ingredients

- 1 small red onion
- 1 red chilli
- 1 lemon
- 2 × 400 g (13 oz) cans cannellini beans
- 3 tablespoons extra virgin olive oil
- 100 g (3½ oz) rocket
- 1 tablespoon olive oil
- 4 tuna steaks
- salt and pepper
- crusty bread, to serve (optional)

Equipment

- kitchen scales
- 1 chopping board
- 1 sharp knife
- 1 grater
- 1 lemon juicer
- can opener
- 1 colander
- 1 mixing bowl
- measuring spoons
- 1 mixing spoon
- 1 griddle pan
- 1 spatula

1. **Clear** your counter of clutter and **set out** all the equipment you need.
2. **Finely slice** the red onion and **deseed** and **chop** the chilli. **Finely grate** the rind of half the lemon, then **juice** the whole lemon.
3. **Drain** and **rinse** the cannellini beans in a colander.
4. **Mix** 2 tablespoons of the lemon juice with the extra virgin olive oil in a mixing bowl and **season** to taste with salt and pepper. **Toss** with the red onion, chilli, cannellini beans, lemon rind and rocket. **Add** more lemon juice if required.
5. **Rub** the olive oil over the tuna steaks and **season** well. **Heat** a griddle pan until smoking hot, then **cook** the tuna over a **high heat** for 1–2 minutes on each side until charred on the outside but still pink in the middle.
6. **Serve** the bean salad with the seared tuna and some crusty bread, if liked.

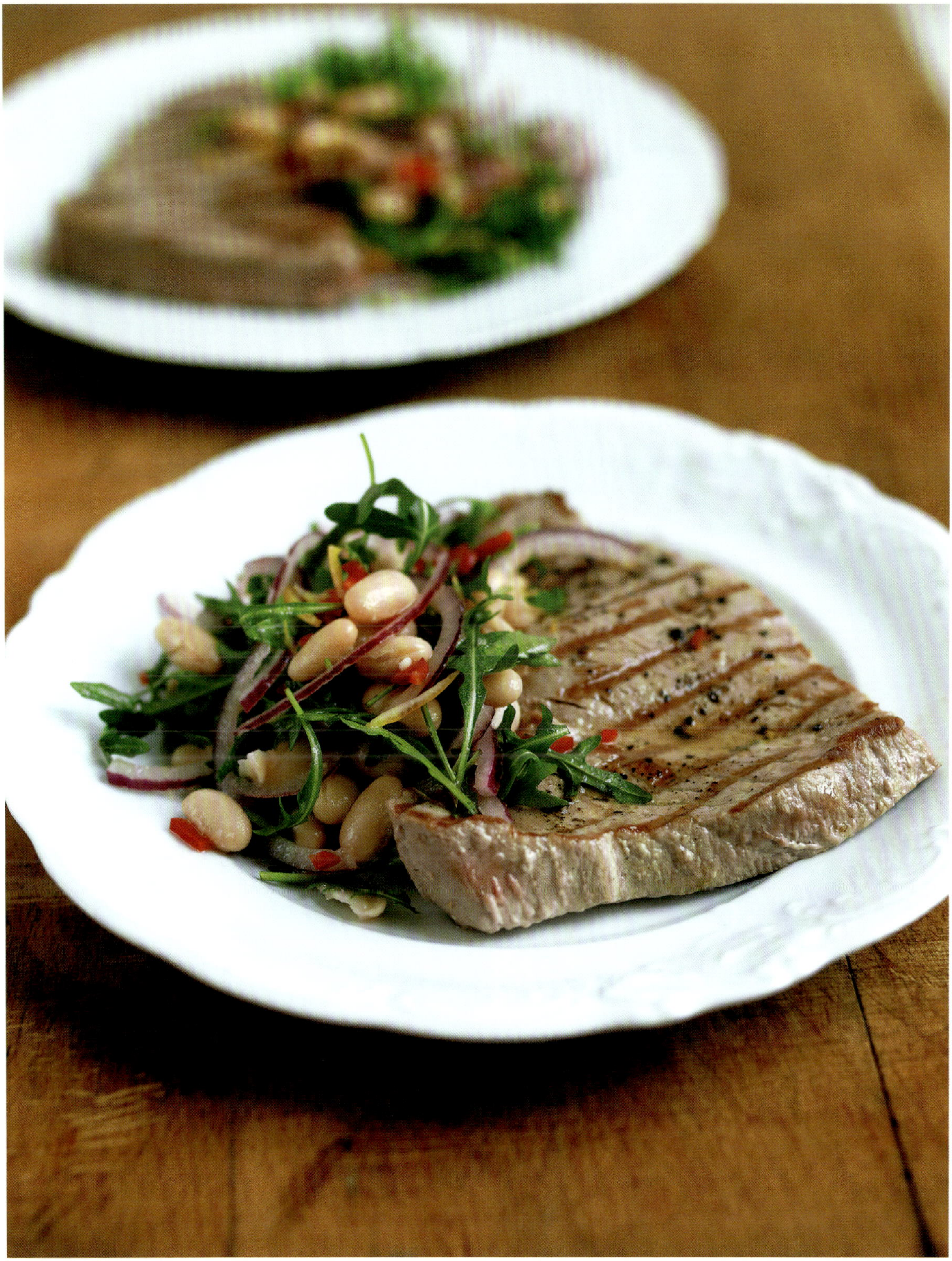

Serves 4 ▪ Preparation time: 10 minutes ▪ Cooking time: 20–25 minutes
Total time: 30–35 minutes

One-pan Sausage Roast

Ingredients

- **1 onion**
- **400 g (13 oz) small new potatoes or new potatoes**
- **2 large carrots**
- **8 Cumberland sausages**
- **2 fresh rosemary sprigs or 1 teaspoon dried rosemary**
- **3 tablespoons olive or vegetable oil**
- **salt and pepper**

Equipment

- **kitchen scales**
- **1 chopping board**
- **1 sharp knife**
- **1 large roasting tin**
- **meaauring spoons**
- **1 wooden spoon**
- **1 spatula**
- **timer**

1. **Clear** your counter of clutter and **set out** all the equipment you need.
2. **Preheat** the oven to **200°C (400°F), Gas Mark 6**.
3. **Cut** the onion into wedges and **halve** the potatoes if small or **cut** into wedges if using (larger) new potatoes. **Cut** the carrots into chunks.
4. **Place** the sausages in a large roasting tin and **add** all the remaining ingredients. **Mix** well to coat everything in the oil and salt and pepper and **spread out** in the tin in a single layer.
5. **Roast** in the oven for 20–25 minutes, **turning** occasionally, until the sausages are cooked and nicely browned and the vegetables are tender. **Set a timer** every 10 minutes to remember to turn the ingredients. **Serve**.

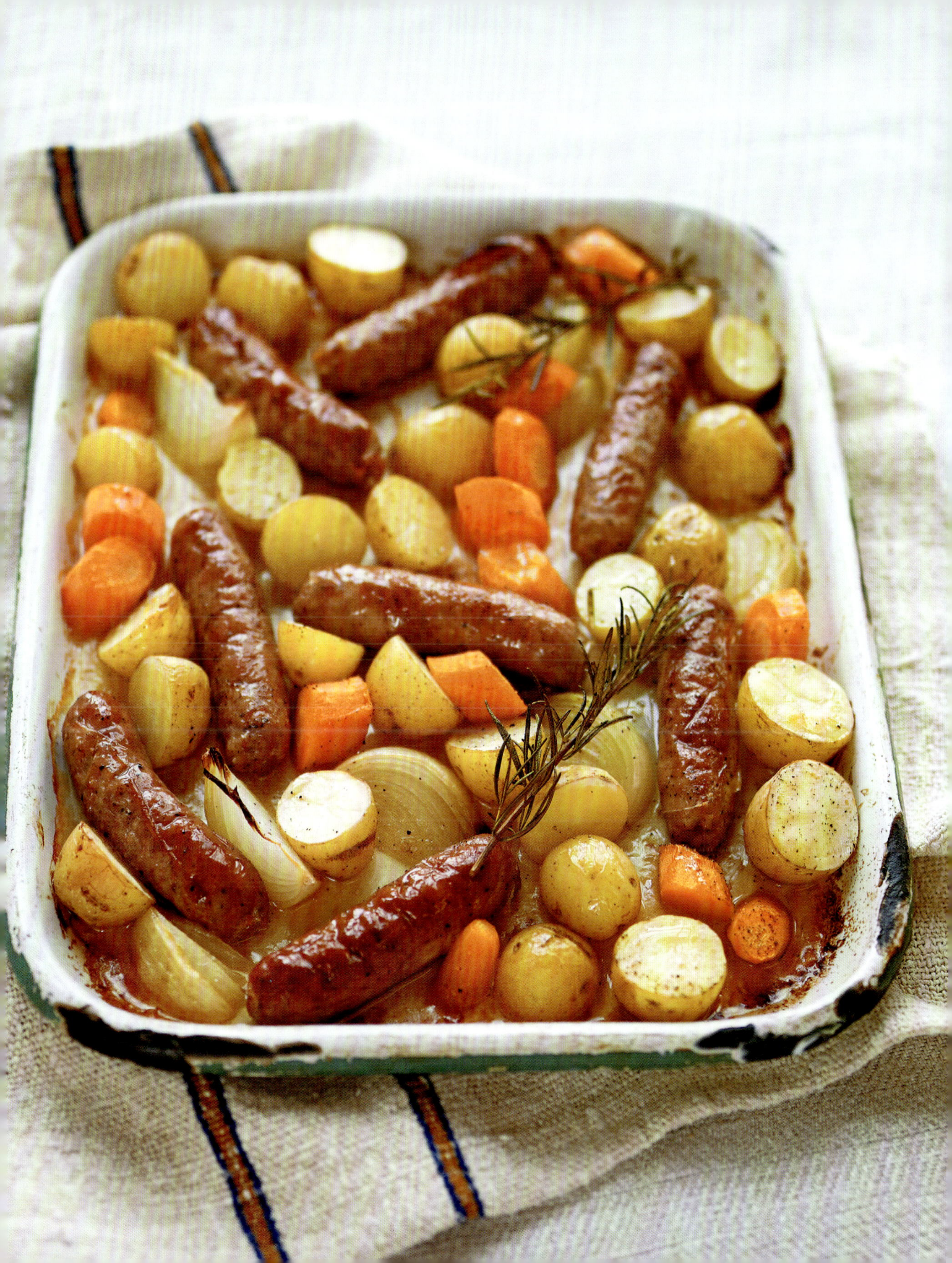

Serves 4 ▪ Preparation time: 10 minutes ▪ Cooking time: 10 minutes
Total time: 20 minutes

Teriyaki Salmon Noodles

Ingredients

- 4 spring onions
- 2.5 cm (1 inch) piece of fresh root ginger
- 375 g (12 oz) dried medium egg noodles
- 3 tablespoons vegetable oil
- 2 × 180 g (6¼ oz) cans skinless, boneless salmon
- 250 g (8 oz) teriyaki stir-fry sauce

Equipment

- kitchen scales
- 1 chopping board
- 1 sharp knife
- 1 saucepan
- can opener
- 1 colander
- measuring spoons
- 1 large frying pan
- 1 wooden spoon
- 1 fork

1. **Clear** your counter of clutter and **set out** all the equipment you need.
2. **Thickly slice** 3 spring onions and **peel** and **cut** the fresh root ginger into matchsticks.
3. **Cook** the noodles in a pan of boiling water for 3–4 minutes or according to the packet instructions until just tender. **Drain** and **toss** in 1 tablespoon of the oil to prevent sticking.
4. **Drain** the salmon.
5. **Heat** the remaining oil in a large frying pan set over a **medium heat** and **cook** the spring onions and ginger for 2–3 minutes until softened and lightly coloured. **Stir** the noodles and the teriyaki stir-fry sauce into the pan and **toss** together to coat.
6. **Flake** over the salmon and **heat** gently for 1–2 minutes until hot.
7. **Heap** into dishes to serve. **Finely slice** the remaining spring onion and **sprinkle** over the top to finish, then **serve**.

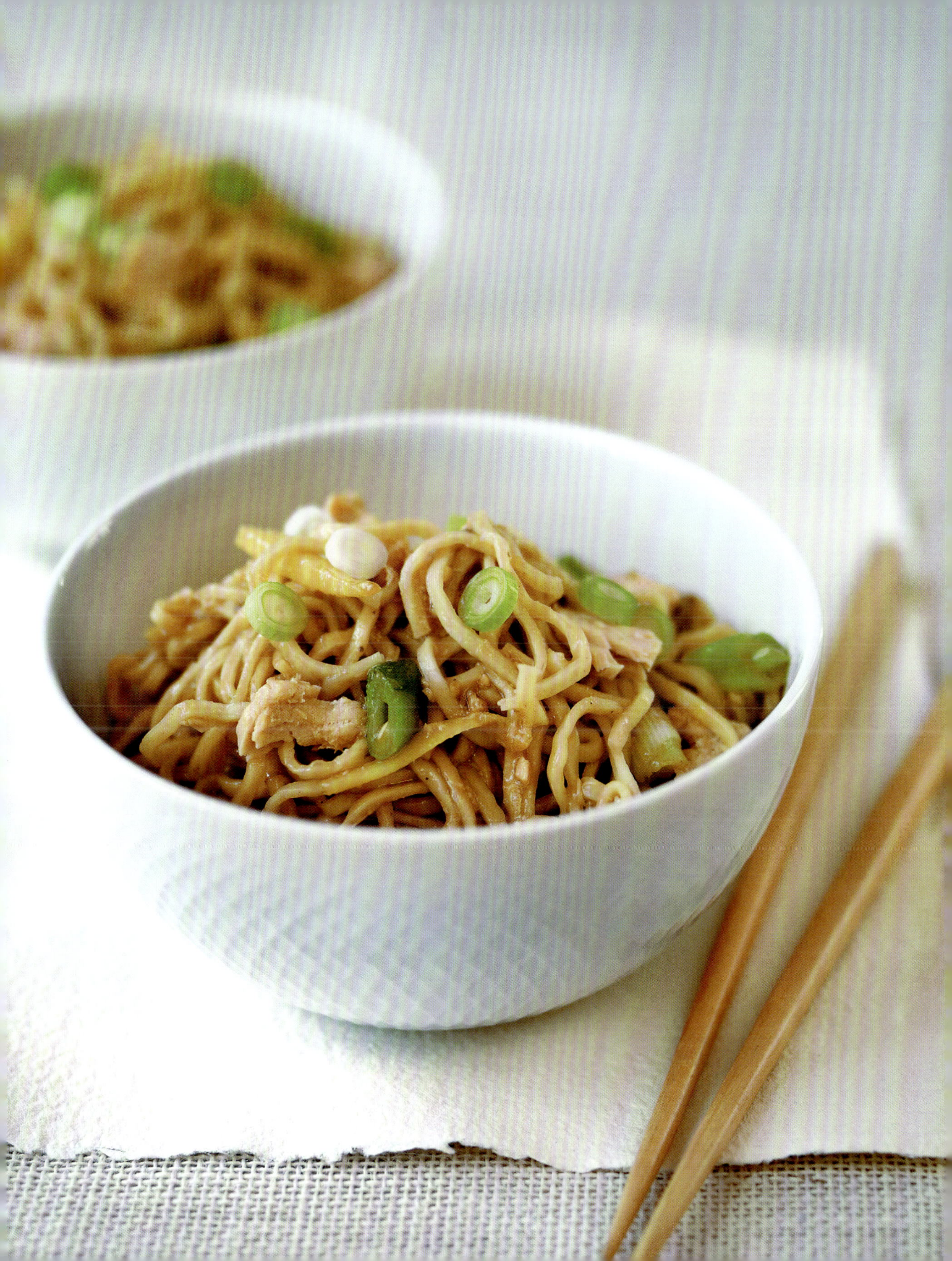

Serves 4 ▪ Preparation time: 15 minutes ▪ Cooking time: 9–13 minutes
Total time: 24–28 minutes

Ginger & Coriander Turkey Burgers

Ingredients

- 10 g (¼ oz) fresh root ginger
- 30 g (1 oz) fresh coriander
- 1 egg
- 450 g (14½ oz) minced turkey
- 50 g (2 oz) fresh breadcrumbs
- 2 teaspoons dark soy sauce
- 2 tablespoons vegetable oil
- 4 large or 8 small bread rolls
- 4 tablespoons chilli jam
- 4–8 lettuce leaves
- pepper

Equipment

- kitchen scales
- 1 chopping board
- 1 vegetable peeler
- 1 grater
- 1 sharp knife
- 1 small bowl or jug
- 1 fork
- 1 large bowl
- measuring spoons
- 1 mixing spoon
- 1 griddle pan
- 1 spatula
- 1 knife

1. **Clear** your counter of clutter and **set out** all the equipment you need.
2. **Peel** and **finely grate** the fresh root ginger and **finely chop** the coriander.
3. **Lightly beat** the egg in a small bowl or jug with a fork.
4. **Place** the minced turkey in a large bowl with the ginger, coriander, breadcrumbs and soy sauce. **Season** with pepper and **add** 2 tablespoons of the beaten egg, **mixing** well to combine. **Shape** into 4 large or 8 small burgers. (**Discard** any leftover egg.)
5. **Brush** a griddle pan with oil and **heat** over a **medium-high heat**. **Griddle** the burgers for 3–4 minutes on each side, until cooked through and nicely browned.
6. **Split** the bread rolls in half and **griddle** for 1–2 minutes on each side.
7. **Spread** the chilli jam on to the bottom halves of the griddled rolls and **top** with the lettuce leaves. **Place** a burger on top of each and **cover** with the roll lid. **Serve** immediately.

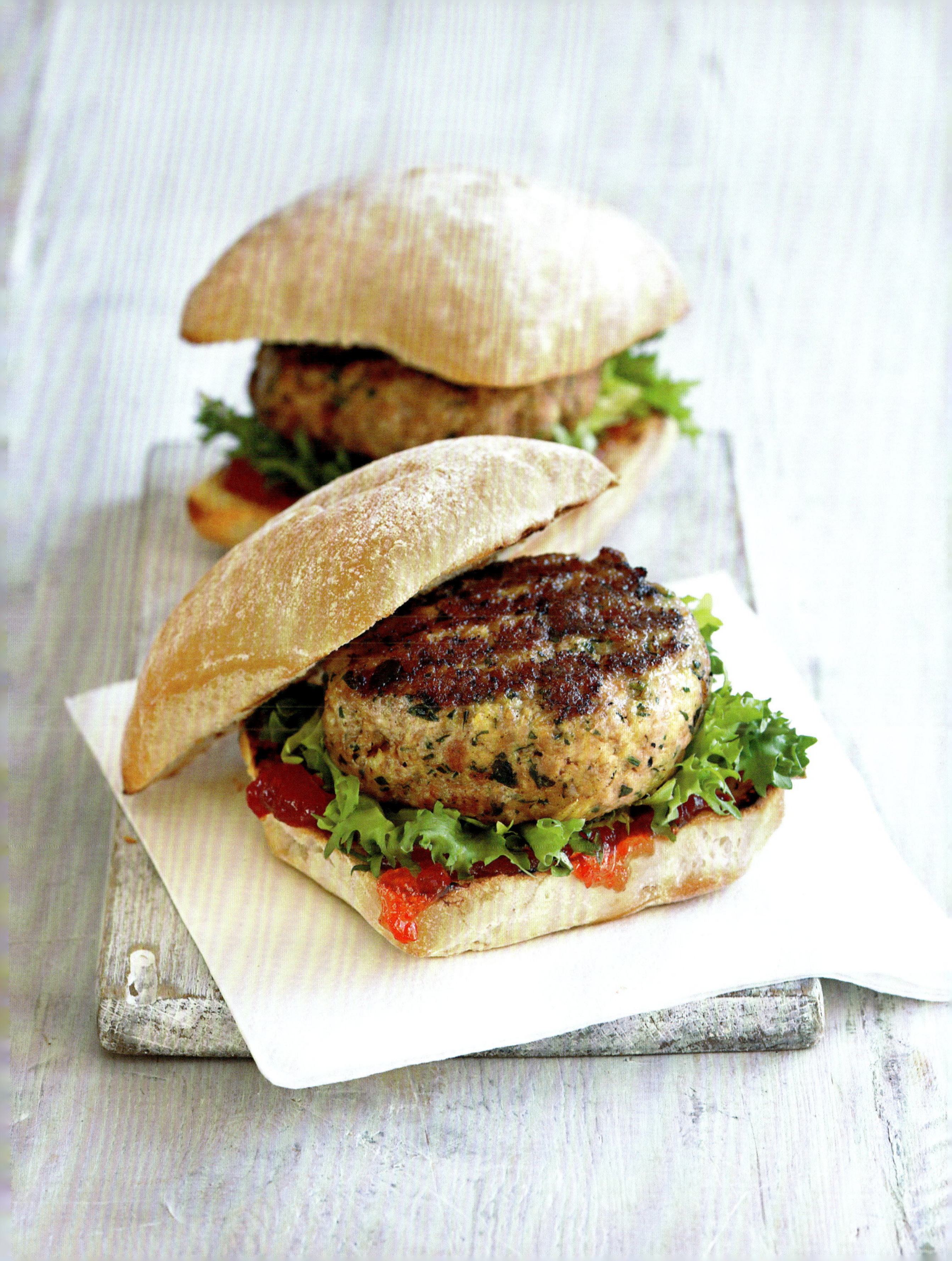

Serves 4 ▪ Preparation time: 10 minutes ▪ Cooking time: 10 minutes
Total time: 20 minutes

Chorizo & Butter Bean Salad

Ingredients

- 1 red onion
- 3 ripe tomatoes
- 30 g (1 oz) fresh parsley
- 100 g (3½ oz) chorizo
- 2 × 400 g (13 oz) cans butter beans
- 2 tablespoons olive or vegetable oil
- 1 teaspoon paprika
- 2 tablespoons sherry or red wine vinegar
- salt and pepper

Equipment

- kitchen scales
- 2 chopping boards
- 2 sharp knives
- can opener
- 1 colander
- 1 large frying pan
- measuring spoons
- 1 wooden spoon

1. **Clear** your counter of clutter and **set out** all the equipment you need.
2. **Finely slice** the red onion. **Chop** the tomatoes and **roughly chop** the parsley.
3. **On a separate chopping board, with a new knife, thinly slice** the chorizo.
4. **Drain** and **rinse** the butter beans in a colander.
5. **Heat** the oil in a large frying pan and **cook** the red onion over a **medium-high heat** for 2–3 minutes, until starting to colour. **Add** the chorizo and **cook** for 1–2 minutes, until golden. **Stir** in the paprika and butter beans and **cook** for a further 1–2 minutes.
6. **Add** the parsley, vinegar and chopped tomatoes to the pan, **toss** well, then **remove** from the heat.
7. **Season** to taste with salt and pepper, then **serve**.

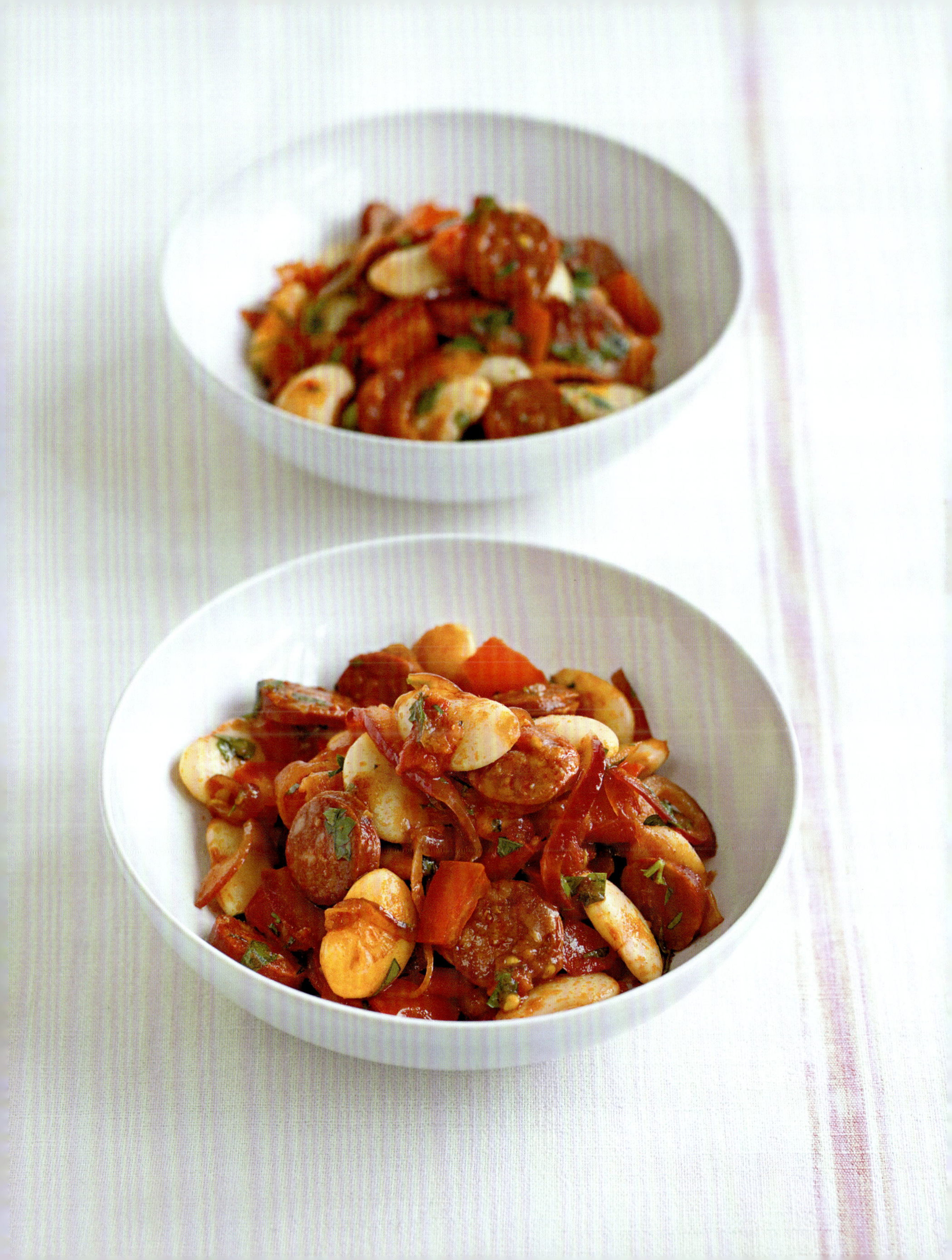

Serves 4 ▪ Preparation time: 10–15 minutes ▪ Cooking time: 30–35 minutes
Total time: 40–50 minutes

Lamb Stew with Feta & Pasta

Ingredients

- **750 ml (1¼ pints) hot chicken stock**
- **400 g (13 oz) lamb fillet or neck**
- **1 onion**
- **1 red pepper**
- **2 garlic cloves**
- **2 tablespoons olive oil**
- **1 tablespoon tomato purée**
- **½ teaspoon ground cinnamon**
- **pinch of dried chilli flakes**
- **300 g (10 oz) dried small soup pasta**
- **25 g (1 oz) feta cheese**
- **salt and pepper**
- **fresh parsley, to garnish**

Equipment

- **kitchen scales**
- **1 measuring jug**
- **2 chopping boards**
- **2 sharp knives**
- **1 large, flameproof casserole dish**
- **measuring spoons**
- **1 wooden spoon**
- **timer**

1. **Clear** your counter of clutter and **set out** all the equipment you need.
2. **Prepare** the stock according to the packet instructions.
3. **Cut** the lamb fillet or neck into bite-sized pieces.
4. **On a separate chopping board, with a new knife, slice** the onion and **core**, **deseed** and **cut** the red pepper into chunks. **Crush** (using the flat side of the knife) and **finely chop** the garlic.
5. **Heat** the oil in a large, flameproof casserole dish. **Add** the lamb and cook on a **medium-high heat** for 5 minutes until starting to brown, then **add** the onion and **cook** for a further 7–8 minutes until soft. **Stir** in the garlic, tomato purée, spices and red pepper, then **pour** in the stock.
6. Bring to the **boil**, then **reduce** the heat and **simmer** for 1–2 minutes. **Add** the pasta and **cook** for 12 minutes, or according to the packet instructions, until the pasta is tender and most of the liquid has boiled away. **Set a timer** every 5 minutes to remind you to give it a **stir**. **Season** to taste with salt and pepper and **crumble** over the feta.
7. **Chop** the parsley, then **sprinkle** it over the pasta to **serve**.

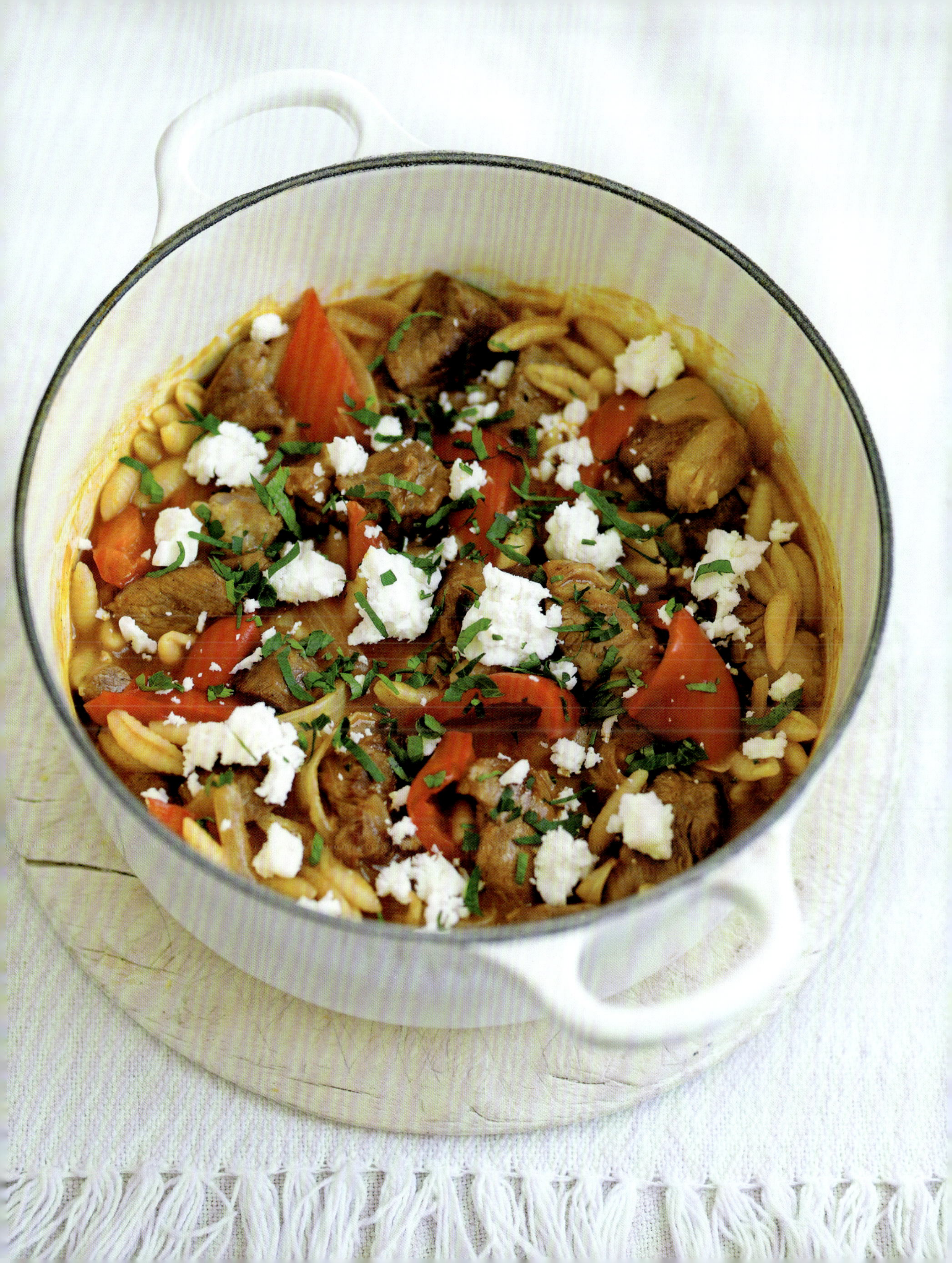

Serves 4 ▪ Preparation time: 15 minutes ▪ Cooking time: 50 minutes
Total time: 1 hour 5 minutes

Masala Dhal with Sweet Potato

Ingredients

- **1 litre (1¾ pints) hot vegetable stock**
- **2 onions**
- **500 g (1 lb) sweet potatoes**
- **2 garlic cloves**
- **1.5 cm (¾ inch) piece of fresh root ginger**
- **250 g (8 oz) dried split yellow peas**
- **3 tablespoons vegetable oil**
- **½ teaspoon dried chilli flakes**
- **2 teaspoons garam masala**
- **½ teaspoon ground turmeric**
- **200 g (7 oz) chopped tomatoes**
- **200 g (7 oz) baby spinach**
- **salt**

Equipment

- **kitchen scales**
- **1 measuring jug**
- **1 chopping board**
- **1 sharp knife**
- **1 vegetable peeler**
- **1 grater**
- **can opener**
- **1 sieve**
- **1 large saucepan with a lid**
- **measuring spoons**
- **1 wooden spoon**
- **timer**

TIP: Serve with mango chutney and warm naan, cooked according to the packet instructions.

1. **Clear** your counter of clutter and **set out** all the equipment you need.
2. **Prepare** the stock according to the packet instructions.
3. **Chop** the onions. **Scrub** the sweet potatoes and **cut** into small chunks. **Crush** (using the flat side of the knife) and **finely chop** the garlic. **Peel** and **grate** the fresh root ginger.
4. **Rinse** and **drain** the split yellow peas.
5. **Heat** the oil in a large saucepan and **fry** the onions over a **medium heat** for 5 minutes. **Add** the garlic, chilli flakes, ginger, garam masala and turmeric and **cook**, **stirring**, for 2 minutes.
6. **Add** the yellow split peas, tomatoes and 750 ml (1¼ pints) of the stock and bring to the **boil**. **Reduce** the heat, **cover** and **cook** gently for 20 minutes until the peas have started to soften. **Set a timer** every 10 minutes to remember to **stir**. **Add** more stock if the mixture runs dry.
7. **Stir** in the sweet potatoes, **re-cover** and **cook** for a further 20 minutes until the potatoes and split peas are tender, **adding** more stock if necessary to keep the dhal juicy. **Tip** the spinach into the pan and **stir** until wilted. **Add** a little salt to taste, then **serve**.

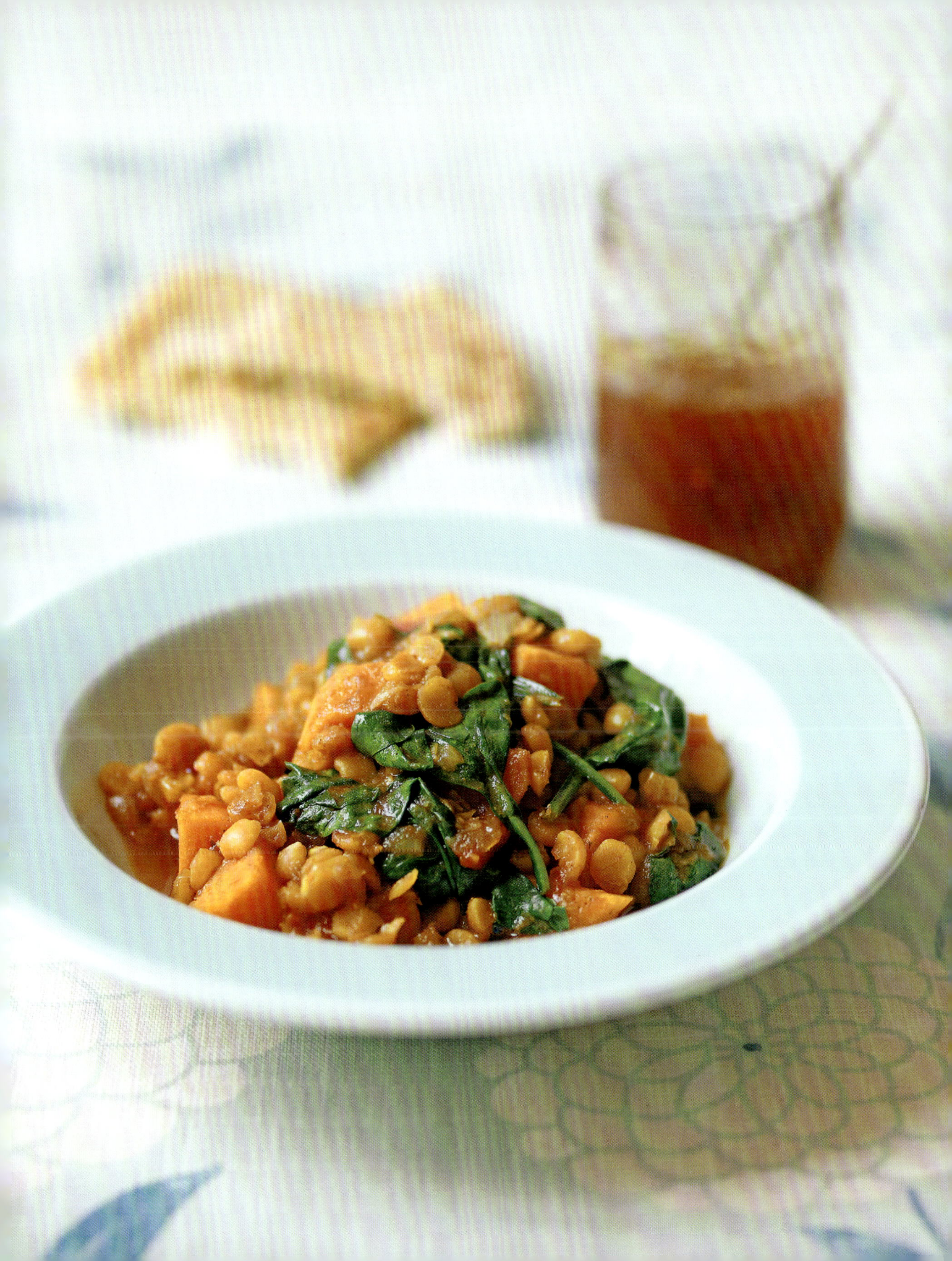

Serves 4 • Preparation time: 10 minutes • Cooking time: 30 minutes
Total time: 40 minutes

Tuna, Spinach & Tomato Penne

Ingredients

- **1 onion**
- **500 g (1 lb) cherry tomatoes**
- **1 garlic clove**
- **2 × 185 g (6½ oz) cans tuna steak in olive oil**
- **2 tablespoons olive oil, plus extra for drizzling**
- **250 g (8 oz) baby spinach**
- **350 g (11½ oz) dried penne**
- **salt and pepper**

Equipment

- **kitchen scales**
- **1 chopping board**
- **1 sharp knife**
- **can opener**
- **2 large saucepans**
- **measuring spoons**
- **1 wooden spoon**
- **1 colander**

1. **Clear** your counter of clutter and **set out** all the equipment you need.
2. **Finely slice** the onion and **halve** the cherry tomatoes. **Crush** (using the flat side of the knife) and **finely chop** the garlic.
3. **Drain** the tuna.
4. **Heat** the oil in a large saucepan, **add** the onion and **fry** gently for 5 minutes, until softened. **Add** the garlic and tomatoes and **fry** for a further 3–4 minutes or until the tomatoes just begin to break up. **Season** with salt and pepper.
5. **Stir** in the spinach, then gently **stir** in the tuna, trying not to break it up too much. **Keep warm** while you cook the pasta.
6. **Cook** the pasta in a large saucepan of salted boiling water according to the packet instructions until al dente.
7. **Drain** the pasta, **add** it to the sauce and **toss** well. **Drizzle** a little more olive oil over the pasta, then **serve**.

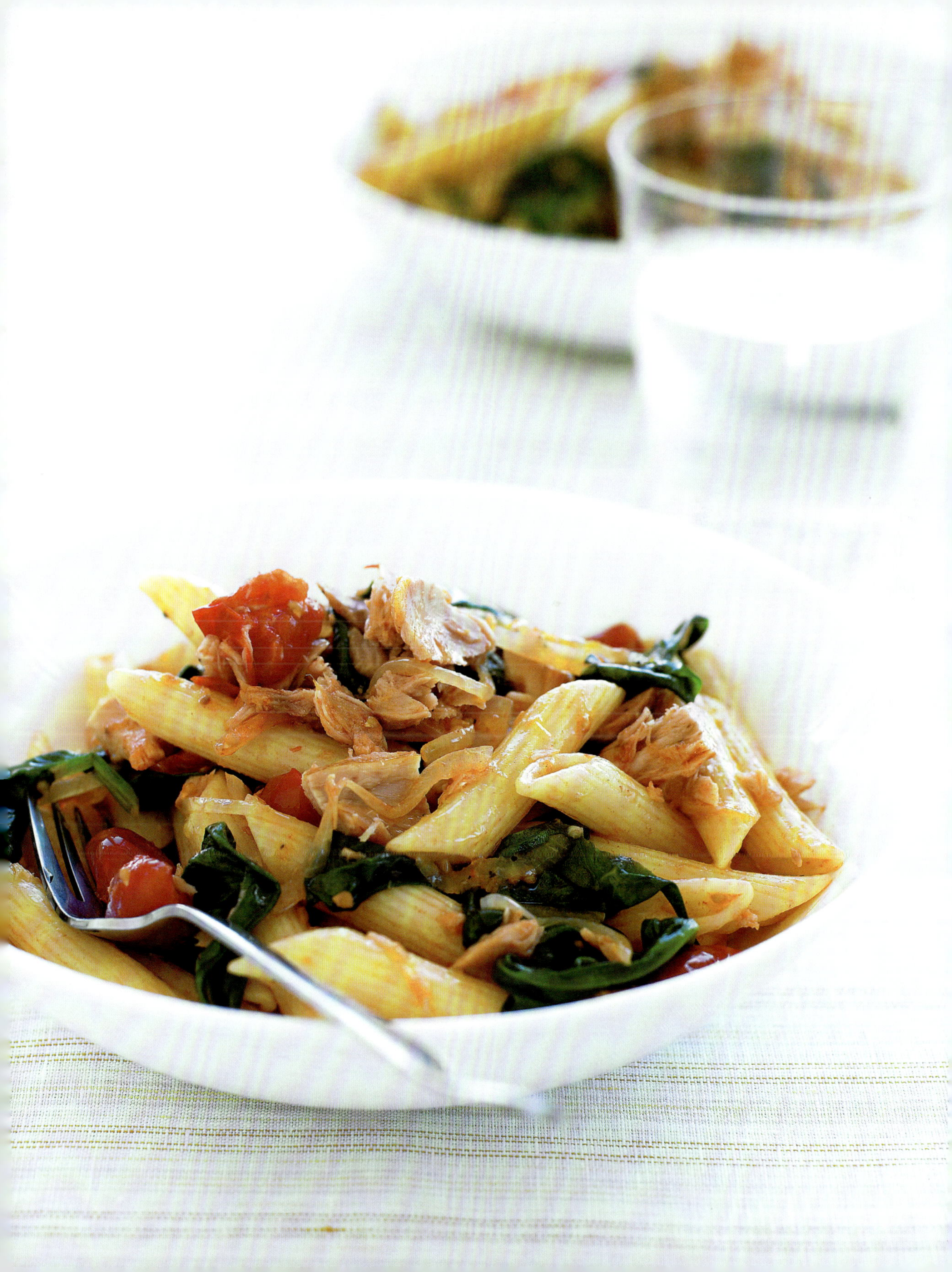

Serves 4 ▪ Preparation time: 25 minutes ▪ Cooking time: 10–12 minutes
Total time: 35–37 minutes

Fresh Tomato Spaghetti

Ingredients

- 750 g (1½ lb) very ripe tomatoes
- 2 garlic cloves
- 10 fresh basil leaves, plus extra to garnish
- 2 teaspoons fennel seeds
- 5 tablespoons extra virgin olive oil
- 2 × 150 g (5 oz) buffalo mozzarella cheese balls
- 400 g (13 oz) dried spaghetti
- salt and pepper

Equipment

- kitchen scales
- 1 chopping board
- 1 knife
- 1 food processor
- 1 large bowl
- measuring spoons
- 1 large saucepan
- 1 colander
- 1 wooden spoon

TIP: Use this as an easy base recipe and add a pre-cooked protein of your choice such as shredded chicken or canned tuna.

1. **Clear** your counter of clutter and **set out** all the equipment you need.
2. **Quarter** the tomatoes and **peel** the garlic. **Put** the tomatoes, garlic and basil in a food processor and **process** until the tomatoes are finely chopped but not smooth. **Transfer** to a large bowl and **add** the fennel seeds and oil. **Season** with salt and pepper. **Leave** the flavours to infuse for at least 15 minutes before cooking the pasta.
3. **Drain**, then **cut** the mozzarella into cubes.
4. **Cook** the spaghetti in a large saucepan of salted boiling water according to the packet instructions until al dente. **Drain**, **stir** into the prepared tomato sauce, then **toss** in the mozzarella.
5. **Serve** immediately, **garnished** with a few extra basil leaves.

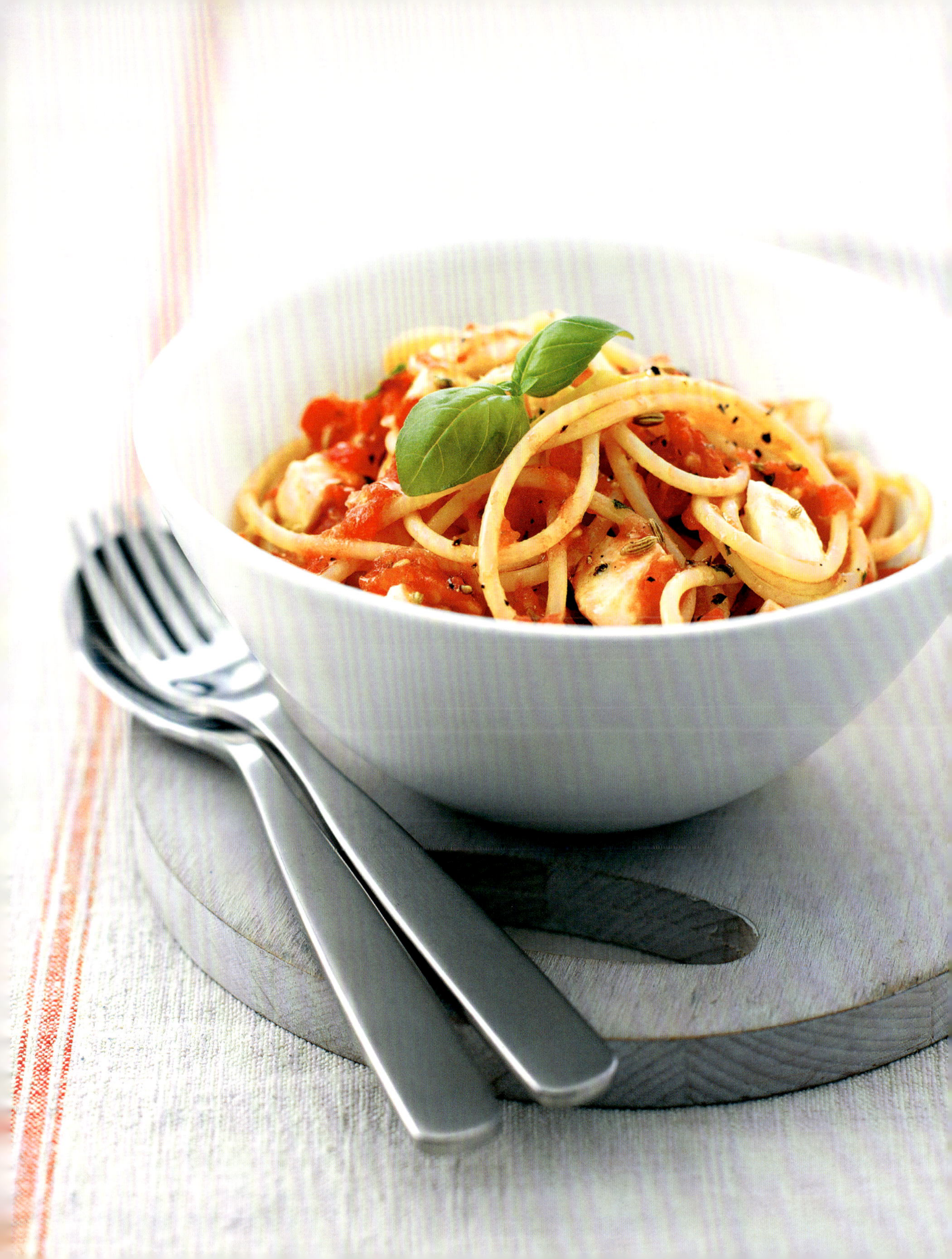

Serves 4 ▪ Preparation time: 10 minutes ▪ Cooking time: 25–30 minutes
Total time: 35–40 minutes

Lentil Bolognese

Ingredients

- 1 onion
- 1 carrot
- 1 celery stick
- 1 garlic clove
- 2 × 400 g (13 oz) cans green lentils
- 3 tablespoons olive oil
- 125 ml (4 fl oz) red wine
- 100 ml (3½ fl oz) water
- 75 g (3 oz) tomato purée
- 400 g (13 oz) can chopped tomatoes
- 1 teaspoon dried mixed herbs
- 50 g (2 oz) Parmesan cheese
- salt and pepper
- crusty bread, to serve

Equipment

- kitchen scales
- measuring jugs
- 1 chopping board
- 1 sharp knife
- can opener
- 1 sieve
- 1 food processor
- 1 large, heavy-based saucepan
- measuring spoons
- 1 wooden spoon
- timer
- 1 grater

1. **Clear** your counter of clutter and **set out** all the equipment you need.
2. **Roughly chop** the onion, carrot and celery. **Peel** the garlic.
3. **Drain** and **rinse** the green lentils.
4. **Place** the onion, carrot, celery and garlic in a food processor and **pulse** briefly until finely chopped.
5. **Heat** the olive oil in a large, heavy-based saucepan. **Add** the vegetable mixture and **cook** over a **medium heat** for 5–6 minutes, **stirring** frequently, until softened and lightly golden.
6. **Pour** in the red wine, measured water, tomato purée, chopped tomatoes and herbs, and **season** to taste with salt and pepper. **Simmer** gently for about 15 minutes, **setting a timer** for every 5 minutes to remember to **stir**.
7. **Add** the lentils and simmer for a further 5–7 minutes, until thickened and tender. **Spoon** into bowls.
8. **Grate** the cheese and **sprinkle** over to **serve**, alongside plenty of fresh crusty bread.

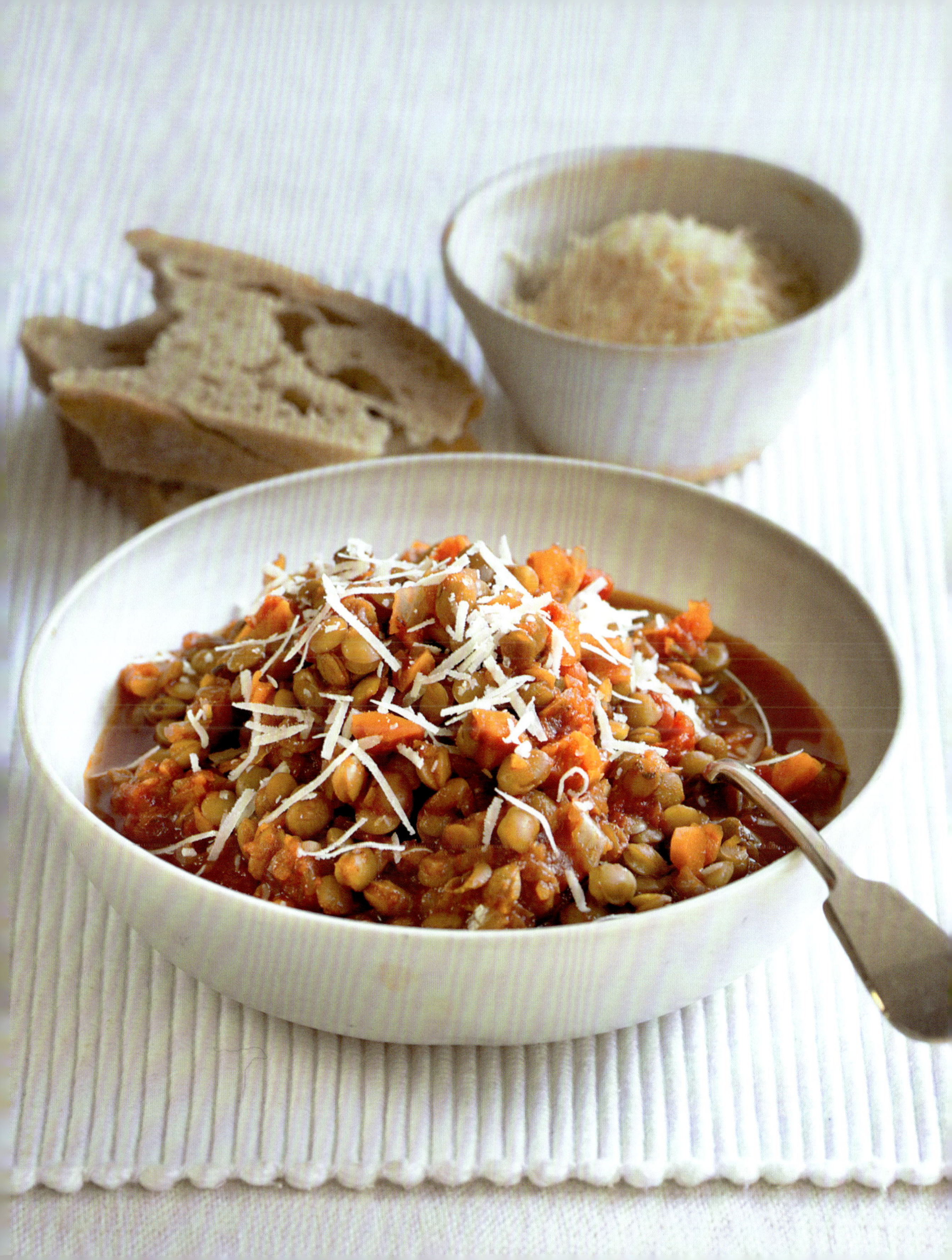

Serves 4 ▪ Preparation time: 15 minutes ▪ Cooking time: 15–20 minutes
Total time: 30–40 minutes

Chicken & Spinach Masala

Ingredients

- **750 g (1½ lb) chicken thighs**
- **1 onion**
- **1 green chilli**
- **300 g (10 oz) spinach**
- **2 garlic cloves**
- **10 g (¼ oz) fresh root ginger**
- **2 tablespoons oil**
- **1 teaspoon ground coriander**
- **1 teaspoon ground cumin**
- **200 g (7 oz) can chopped tomatoes**
- **200 ml (7 fl oz) crème fraîche**
- **20 g (¾ oz) fresh coriander**
- **salt and pepper**
- **flatbreads, to serve**

Equipment

- **kitchen scales**
- **1 measuring jug**
- **2 chopping boards**
- **2 sharp knives**
- **1 vegetable peeler**
- **1 grater**
- **1 large, heavy-based saucepan with a lid**
- **measuring spoons**
- **1 wooden spoon**
- **can opener**

1. **Clear** your counter of clutter and **set out** all the equipment you need.
2. **Skin**, **bone** and **cut** the chicken thighs into bite-sized chunks.
3. **On a separate chopping board, with a new knife**, **thinly slice** the onion. **Deseed** and **thinly slice** the chilli and **roughly chop** the spinach. **Crush** (using the flat side of the knife) and **finely chop** the garlic. **Peel** and **finely grate** the fresh root ginger.
4. **Heat** the oil in a large, heavy-based saucepan. **Add** the onion, garlic, chilli and ginger. **Stir-fry** over a **medium-high heat** for 2–3 minutes and then **add** the ground coriander and cumin. **Stir** and **cook** for a further 1 minute.
5. **Pour** in the tomatoes and **cook** gently for 3 minutes. **Increase the heat** and **add** the chicken. **Cook**, **stirring**, until the outside of the chicken is sealed. **Stir** in the crème fraîche and spinach.
6. **Cover** the pan and **cook** the chicken mixture gently for 6–8 minutes, **stirring** occasionally.
7. **Chop** the fresh coriander and **stir** it in. **Season** to taste with salt and pepper and **serve** with the flatbreads.

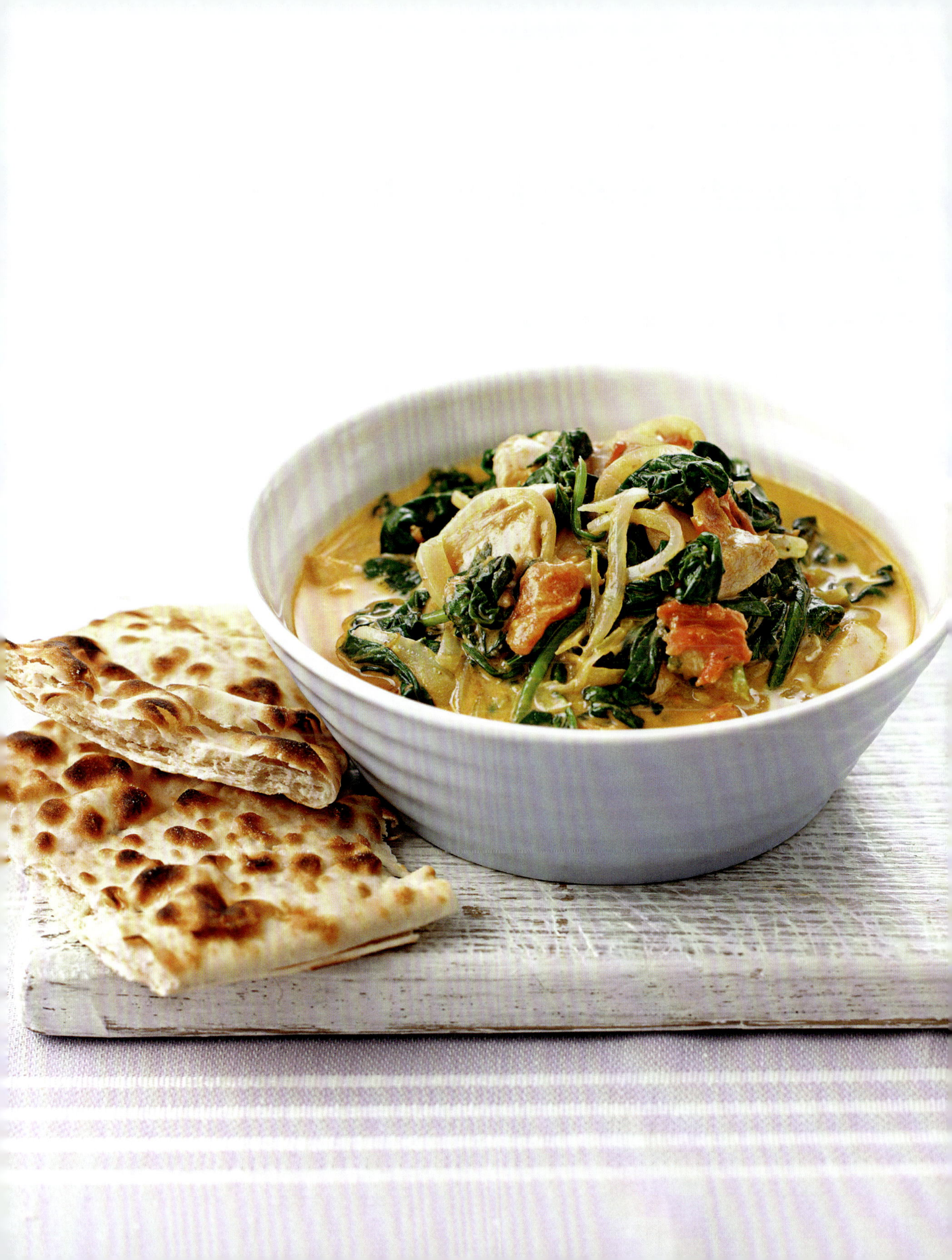

Serves 4 ▪ Preparation time: 10 minutes ▪ Cooking time: 12–17 minutes
Total time: 22–27 minutes

Thai-style Monkfish & Prawn Curry

Ingredients

- **300 g (10 oz) monkfish or cod loins**
- **50 g (2 oz) green beans**
- **1 lime**
- **3 tablespoons Thai green curry paste**
- **400 ml (14 fl oz) can coconut milk**
- **2 makrut lime leaves (fresh or dried, optional)**
- **1 tablespoon soft brown sugar**
- **12 raw peeled tiger prawns**
- **2–3 tablespoons Thai fish sauce**
- **1–2 green chillies**
- **fresh coriander sprigs**
- **microwave rice, to serve**

Equipment

- **kitchen scales**
- **2 chopping boards**
- **2 sharp knives**
- **1 lemon juicer**
- **measuring spoons**
- **can opener**
- **1 saucepan**
- **1 rolling pin**
- **1 wooden spoon**

1. **Clear** your counter of clutter and **set out** all the equipment you need.
2. **Cut** the monkfish or cod into cubes.
3. **On a separate chopping board, with a new knife**, **halve** the lemon grass stalk, if using, lengthways and **trim** and **halve** the green beans. **Halve** and **juice** the lime.
4. **Put** the curry paste and coconut milk in a saucepan. **Add** the lime leaves, if using, and the sugar. Bring to the **boil**, then **add** the monkfish or cod. **Simmer** gently for 2 minutes, then **add** the green beans and **cook** for a further 2 minutes or until the fish is cooked through.
5. **Stir** in the prawns, fish sauce and 2 tablespoons of the lime juice and **cook** for 2–5 minutes until the prawns turn pink and are cooked through.
6. **Microwave** the rice according to the packet instructions.
7. **Transfer** the curry to warm serving dishes. **Slice** the chillies and **sprinkle** over the curry along with the coriander sprigs, then **serve** with the rice.

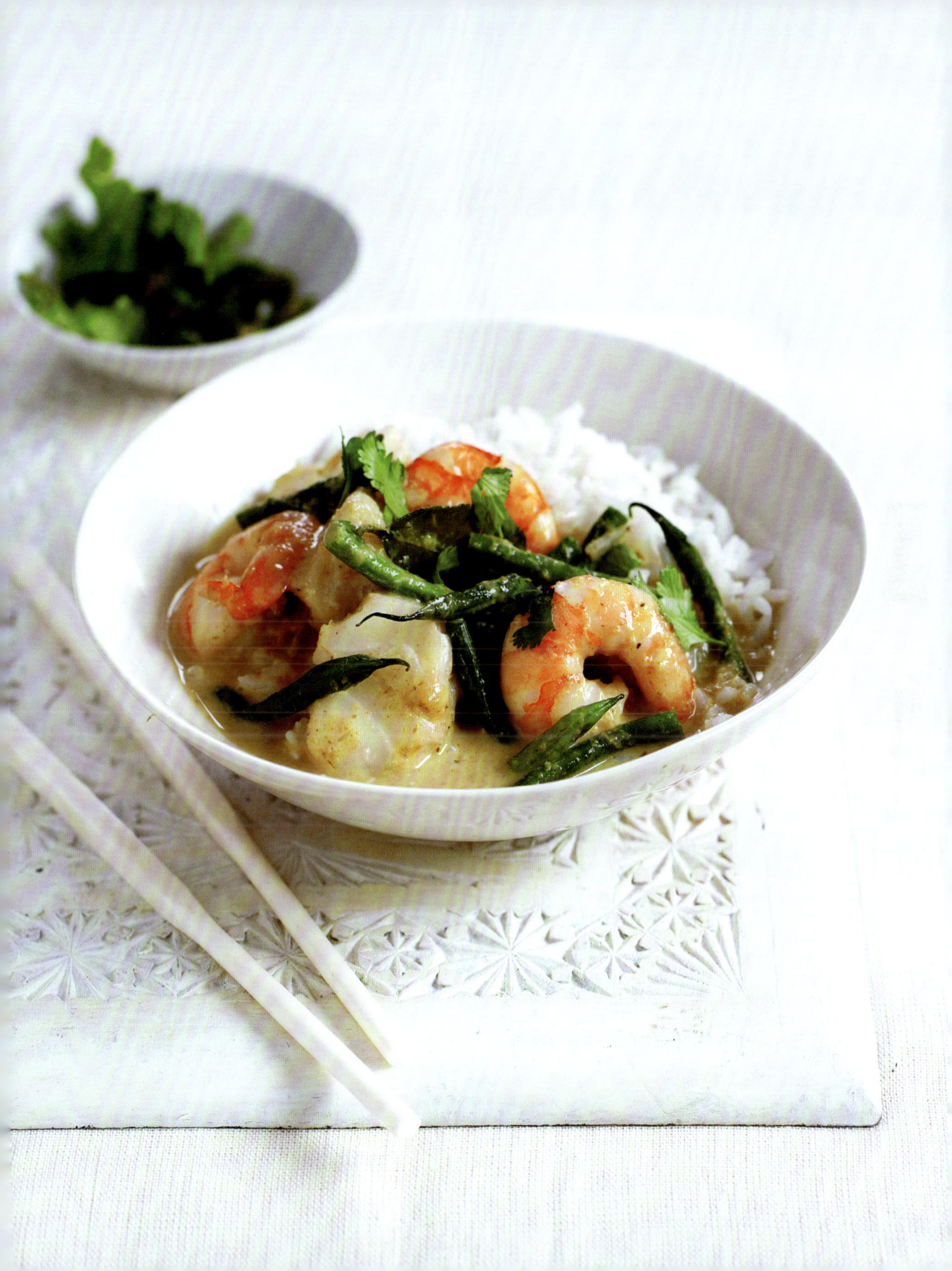

Serves 4 ▪ Preparation time: 5 minutes ▪ Cooking time: 30 minutes
Total time: 35 minutes

Pasta Puttanesca

Ingredients

- 2 garlic cloves
- 8 anchovy fillets in oil
- 1 tablespoon capers
- 3 tablespoons olive oil
- ½ teaspoon dried chilli flakes
- 2 × 400 g (13 oz) cans chopped tomatoes
- 125 g (4 oz) black olives
- 300 g (10 oz) dried pappardelle
- salt and pepper
- fresh basil leaves, to garnish

Equipment

- kitchen scales
- 1 chopping board
- 1 sharp knife
- can opener
- 2 large saucepans
- measuring spoons
- 1 wooden spoon
- timer
- 1 colander

1. **Clear** your counter of clutter and **set out** all the equipment you need.
2. **Slice** the garlic. **Drain** the anchovies and **drain** and **rinse** the capers.
3. **Heat** the oil in a large saucepan, add the garlic, chilli flakes and anchovies and **cook** over a **high heat**, **stirring** frequently, for a couple of minutes until the anchovies begin to disintegrate.
4. **Stir** in the tomatoes and **cook**, fairly vigorously, for 15 minutes or until the sauce has thickened. **Set a timer** every 5 minutes to remind you to give it a **stir**. **Add** the olives and capers and **season** with salt and pepper. **Keep warm** while you cook the pasta.
5. **Cook** the pappardelle in a large saucepan of salted boiling water according to the packet instructions until al dente. **Drain** and then **toss** through the sauce.
6. **Spoon** into serving bowls and **tear** over the basil leaves.

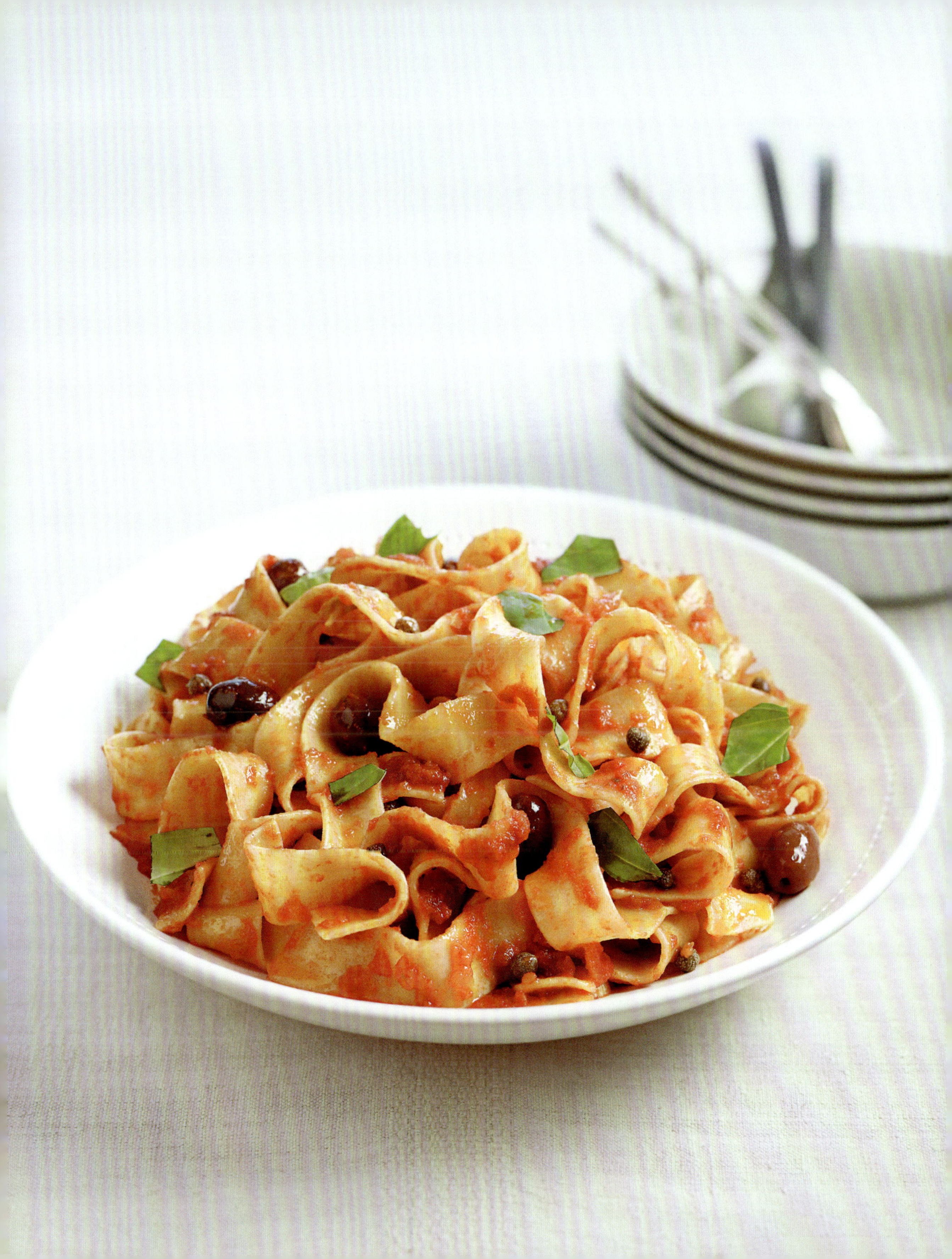

Serves 4–6 ▪ Preparation time: 1 hour 15 minutes ▪ Cooking time: None
Total time: 1 hour 15 minutes

Bulgur Wheat Salad

Ingredients

- **150 g (5 oz) bulgur wheat**
- **1 lemon**
- **¼ teaspoon ground allspice**
- **¼ teaspoon ground cinnamon**
- **4 tablespoons olive oil**
- **400 g (13 oz) cherry tomatoes**
- **6 spring onions**
- **bunch of fresh parsley**
- **small bunch of fresh mint**
- **salt and pepper**

Equipment

- **kitchen scales**
- **2 bowls**
- **1 lemon juicer**
- **measuring spoons**
- **1 fork or whisk**
- **1 fine sieve**
- **1 chopping board**
- **1 sharp knife**
- **1 mixing spoon**

TIP: Make a batch of this at the beginning of the week and add a ready-cooked protein of your choice when serving, such as shredded chicken or canned tuna.

1. **Clear** your counter of clutter and **set out** all the equipment you need.
2. **Put** the bulgar wheat in a bowl and **cover** with cold water. **Leave to soak** for at least 1 hour.
3. To make the dressing, **halve** and **juice** the lemon and **whisk** the juice together with the allspice, cinnamon and oil.
4. **Strain** the bulgur wheat through a fine sieve and **leave to stand** for 5 minutes, **squeezing** out as much water as possible.
5. **Halve** the cherry tomatoes and **finely chop** the spring onions. **Chop** the parsley and mint.
6. **Add** the tomatoes, spring onions, parsley and mint to the bulgur wheat. **Add** the dressing and **mix** well. **Season** with salt and pepper to taste. Leaving the salad in the refrigerator for a few hours before serving will intensify the flavours.

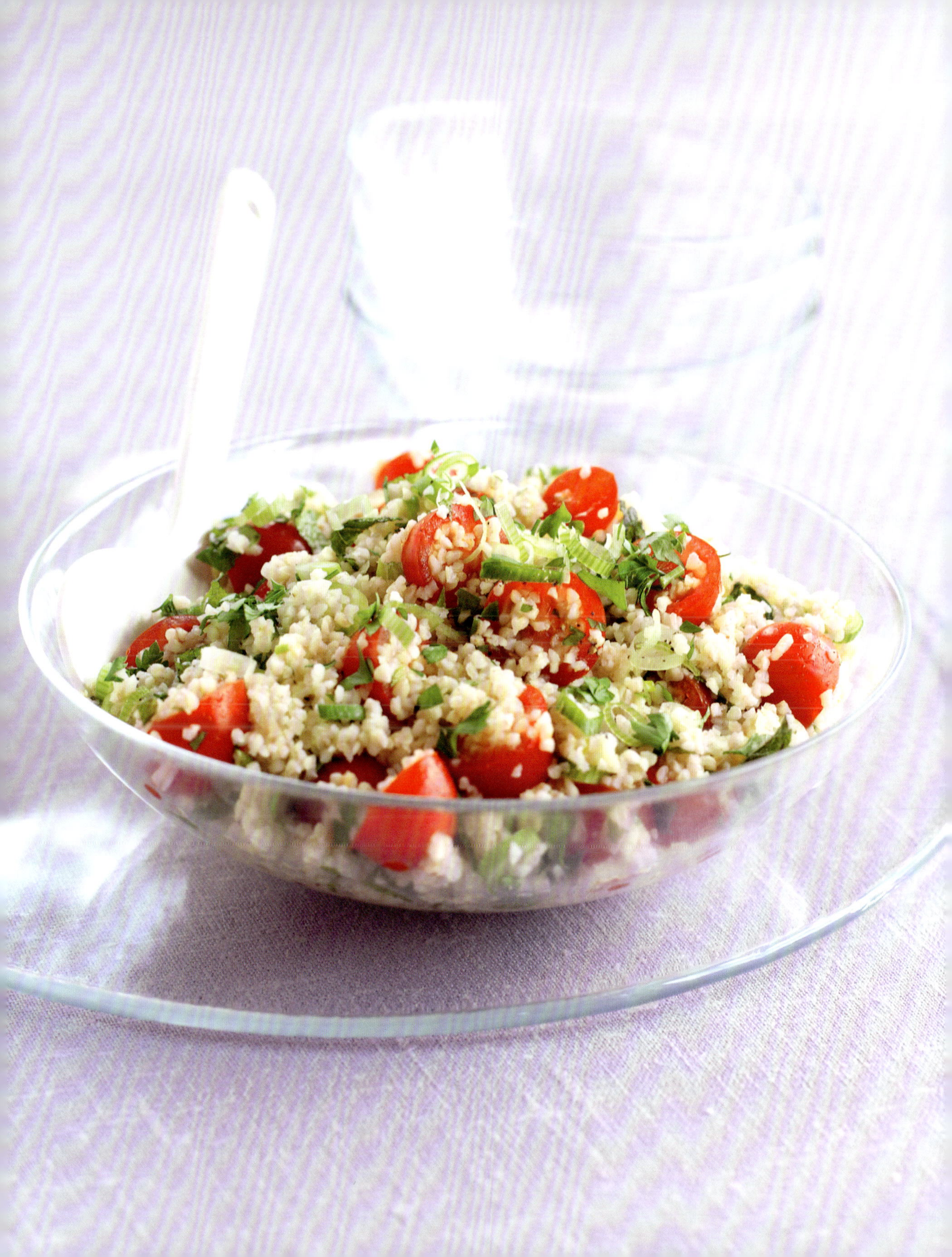

Serves 4 ▪ Preparation time: 10 minutes ▪ Cooking time: 20–25 minutes
Total time: 30–35 minutes

Roasted Chicken with Butternut Squash

Ingredients

- **500 g (1 lb) butternut squash**
- **1 red onion**
- **4 bone-in, skin-on chicken breasts**
- **2 tablespoons olive oil**
- **1 tablespoon balsamic vinegar**
- **25 g (1 oz) walnut halves**
- **8 fresh sage leaves**
- **salt and pepper**
- **green salad, to serve**

Equipment

- **kitchen scales**
- **1 vegetable peeler**
- **1 chopping board**
- **1 sharp knife**
- **1 roasting tin**
- **measuring spoon**
- **1 mixing spoon**

1. **Clear** your counter of clutter and **set out** all the equipment you need.
2. **Preheat** the oven to **200°C (400°F), Gas Mark 6**.
3. **Peel** the butternut squash, then **deseed** and **cut** into thin slices. **Slice** the red onion.
4. **Arrange** the squash, red onion and chicken breasts, skin side up, in a roasting tin.
5. **Drizzle** over the oil, **season** to taste with salt and pepper and **toss** to make sure everything is well coated in oil. **Roast** in the oven for 15 minutes.
6. **Drizzle** over the balsamic vinegar and **scatter** the walnuts and sage leaves around the chicken. **Return** to the oven for 5–10 minutes until the squash is tender and the chicken is cooked through.
7. **Serve** with a green salad.

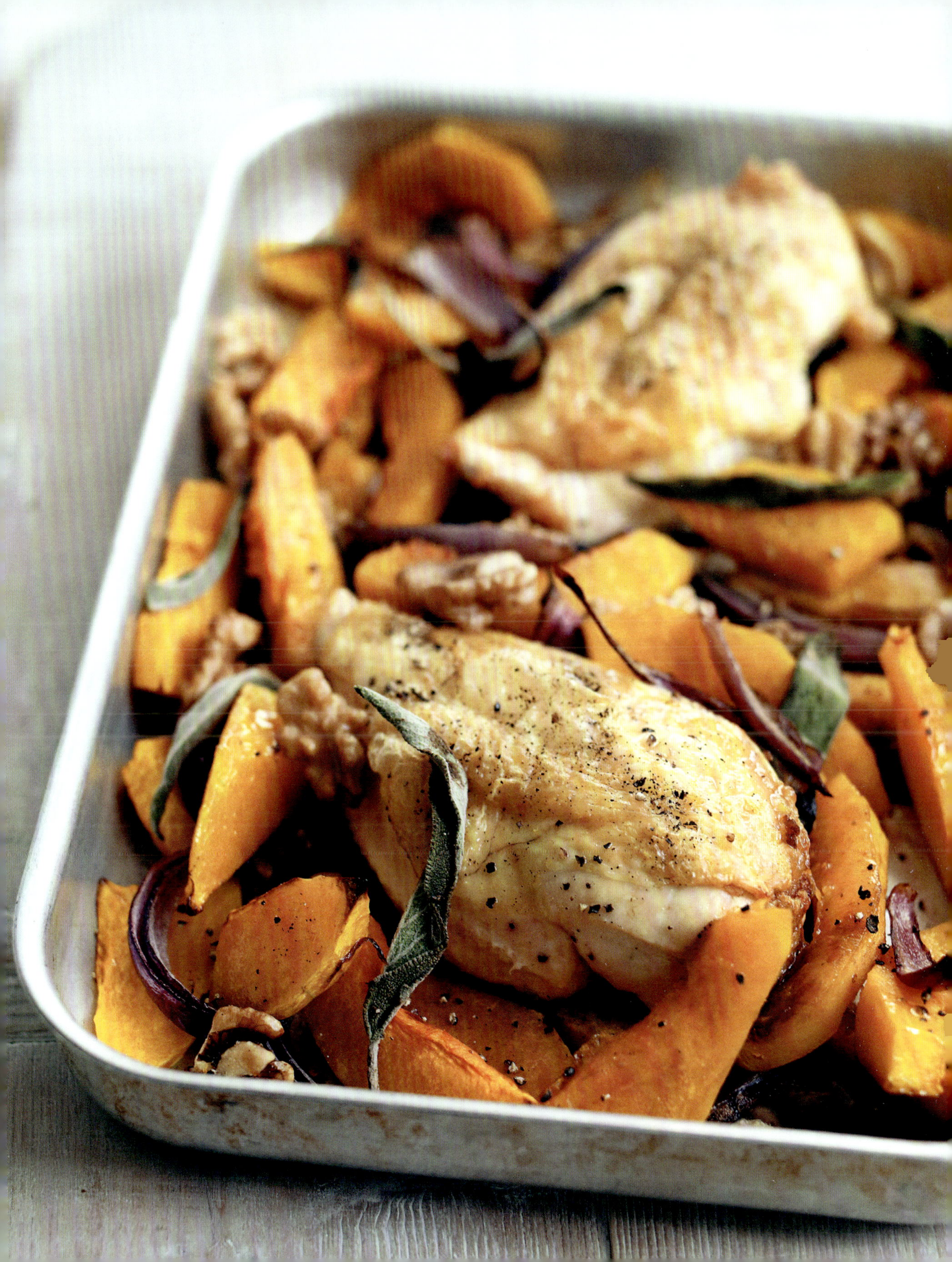

Serves 4 ▪ Preparation time: 10 minutes ▪ Cooking time: 25–30 minutes
Total time: 35–40 minutes

Pork & Tomato Rice Pot

Ingredients

- 650 ml (1 pint 2 fl oz) hot chicken stock
- 300 g (10 oz) pork fillet
- 1 onion
- 3 garlic cloves
- 3 tablespoons olive oil
- 250 g (8 oz) paella rice
- 2 teaspoons smoked paprika
- 200 g (7 oz) can chopped tomatoes
- 125 g (4 oz) baby spinach
- salt and pepper
- 1 lemon, to serve

Equipment

- kitchen scales
- 1 measuring jug
- 2 chopping boards
- 2 sharp knives
- 1 large, deep frying pan with a lid
- 1 plate
- measuring spoons
- 1 wooden spoon
- can opener
- timer
- 1 fork

1. **Clear** your counter of clutter and **set out** all the equipment you need.
2. **Prepare** the stock according to the packet instructions.
3. **Slice** the pork fillet.
4. **On a separate chopping board, with a new knife, finely chop** the onion and garlic.
5. **Heat** 1 tablespoon of the oil in a large, deep frying pan over a **high heat**, **add** the pork and **cook** for 3 minutes until golden and almost cooked through. **Remove** from the pan to a plate and **set aside**.
6. **Add** the remaining oil to the pan, **reduce** the heat to **medium** and **cook** the onion for 3 minutes until softened, then **stir** in the garlic and **cook** for a further 30 seconds. **Add** the rice and **cook** for 1 minute, then **add** the paprika and tomatoes.
7. Bring to the **boil**, then **reduce** the heat and **simmer** for 2–3 minutes. **Pour** in the stock, **season** with salt and pepper and **cook** for a further 12–15 minutes until most of the liquid has been absorbed. **Set a timer** every 5 minutes to remind you to give it a **stir**.
8. **Fork** the spinach through the rice, **arrange** the pork on top, then **cover** and continue to **cook** for 3–4 minutes until cooked through.
9. **Cut** the lemon into wedges and **serve** alongside the rice.

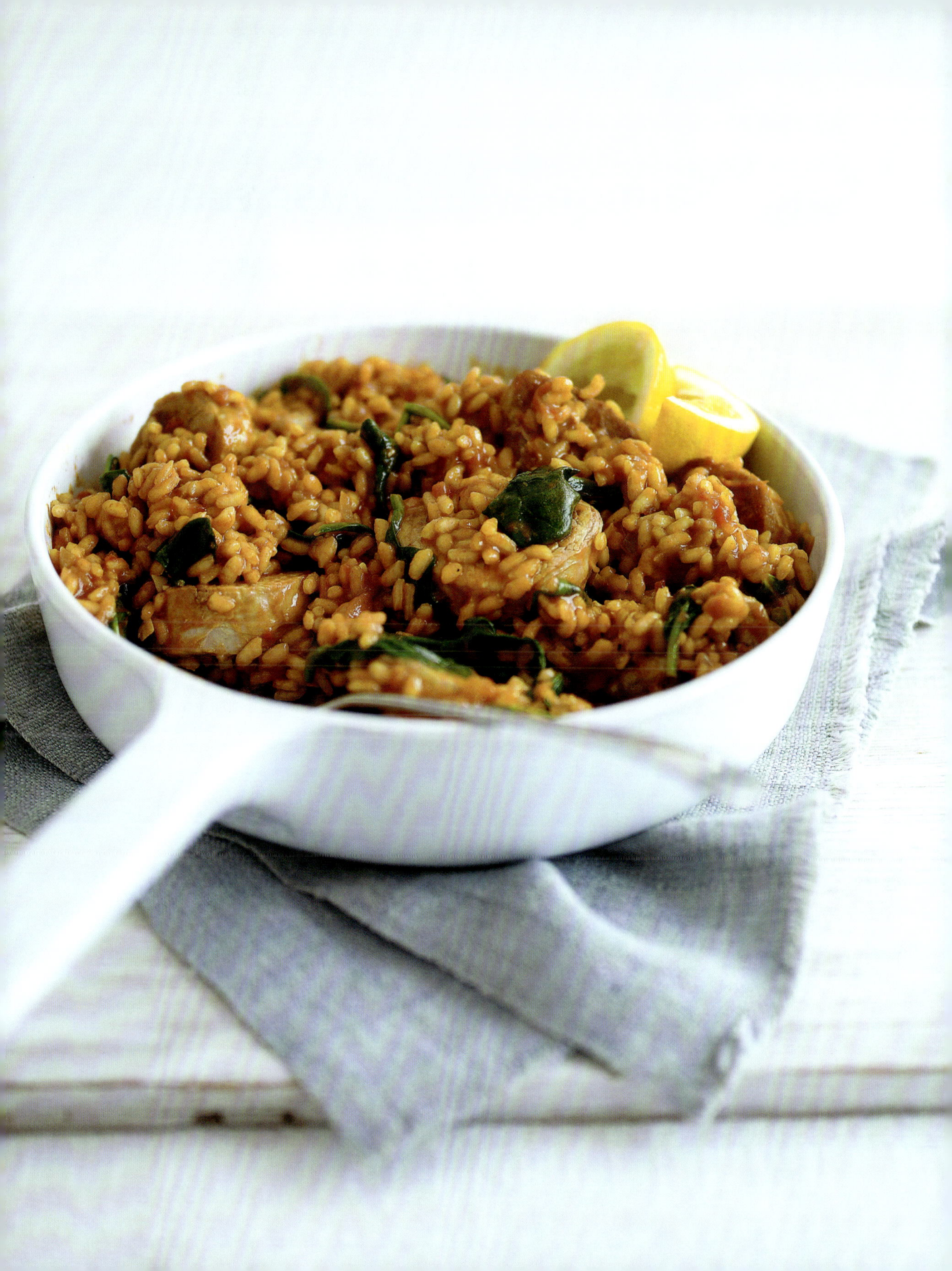

Serves 4 ▪ Preparation time: 10 minutes ▪ Cooking time: 18 minutes
Total time: 28 minutes

Spicy Salmon with Couscous

Ingredients

- **325 ml (11 fl oz) hot chicken or fish stock**
- **1 tablespoon olive oil, plus extra for greasing**
- **1 lemon**
- **1 teaspoon ground cumin**
- **½ teaspoon ground coriander**
- **pinch of dried chilli flakes**
- **4 skinless salmon fillets**
- **2 teaspoons clear honey**
- **300 g (10 oz) couscous**
- **2 spring onions**
- **handful of fresh coriander**
- **25 g (1 oz) toasted flaked almonds**
- **salt and pepper**

Equipment

- **kitchen scales**
- **1 small roasting tin**
- **1 measuring jug**
- **1 grater**
- **1 mixing bowl**
- **measuring spoons**
- **foil**
- **1 chopping board**
- **1 sharp knife**

1. **Clear** your counter of clutter and **set out** all the equipment you need.
2. **Preheat** the oven to **200°C (400°F), Gas Mark 6**. **Lightly grease** a small roasting tin.
3. **Prepare** the stock according to the packet instructions.
4. **Finely grate** the lemon rind. **Add** to a bowl with the measured oil, spices and lemon rind, **mix** to combine, then **rub** all over the salmon fillets. **Season** to taste with salt and pepper and **arrange** in the prepared roasting tin.
5. **Cook** the salmon in the oven for 10 minutes, then **drizzle** over the honey and **return** to the oven for a further 3 minutes until golden and cooked through.
6. **Remove** from the oven, **scatter** the couscous around the salmon and **pour** in the stock. **Cover** tightly with foil and **leave** for 5 minutes until the couscous is tender.
7. **Transfer** the salmon to plates.
8. **Slice** the spring onions and **chop** the coriander, then **stir** these into the couscous with the toasted flaked almonds. **Serve** with the salmon.

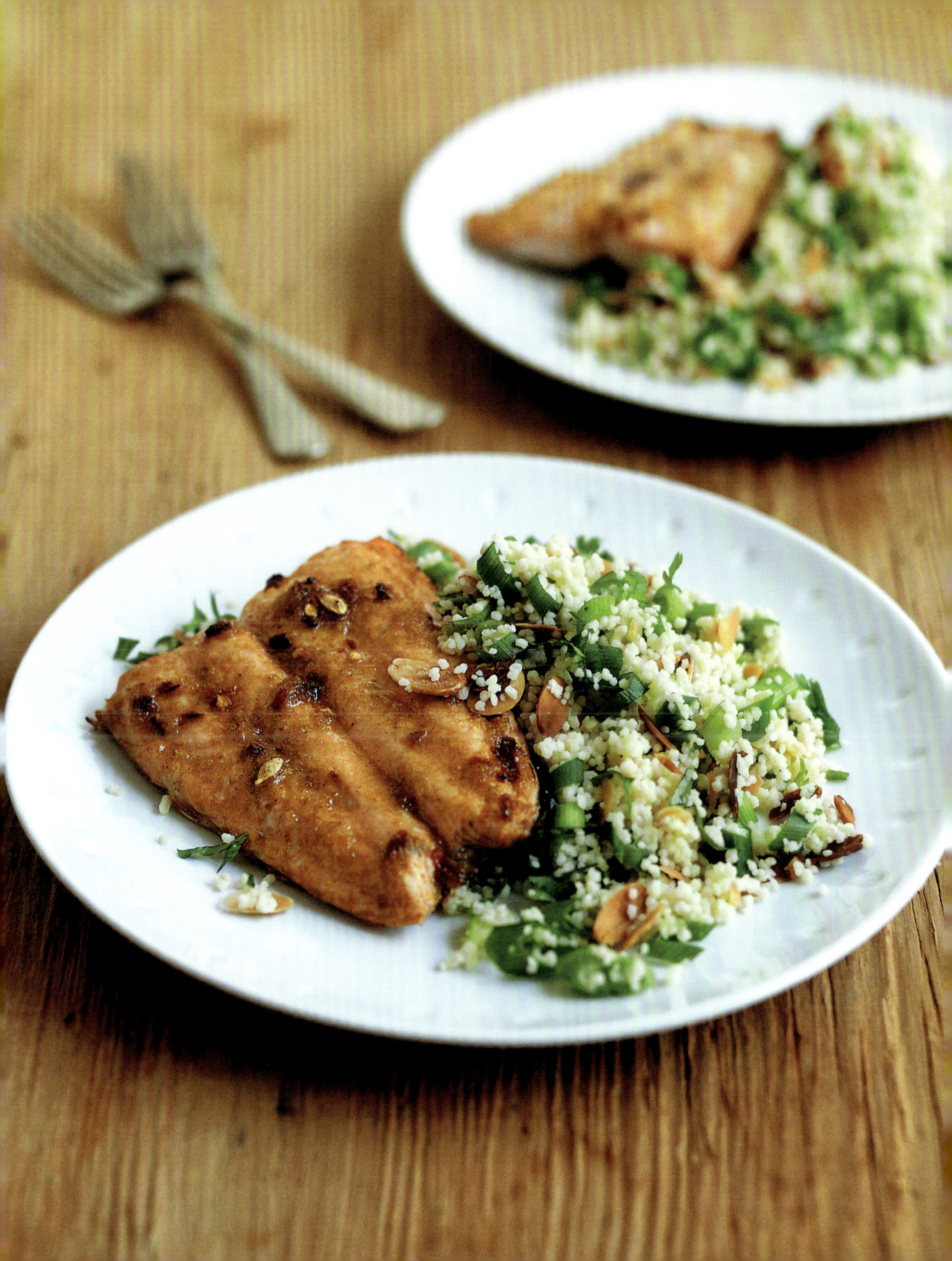

Serves 4 ▪ Preparation time: 10 minutes ▪ Cooking time: 20 minutes
Total time: 30 minutes

Sausage & Bean Casserole

Ingredients

- **150 ml (¼ pint) hot vegetable stock**
- **8 lean pork sausages, about 500 g (1 lb) in total**
- **1 onion**
- **1 red pepper**
- **1 garlic clove**
- **2 × 410 g (13½ oz) cans mixed beans**
- **1 tablespoon oil**
- **400 g (13 oz) can chopped tomatoes**
- **2 tablespoons tomato purée**
- **20 g (¾ oz) fresh parsley**
- **salt and pepper**

Equipment

- **kitchen scales**
- **1 measuring jug**
- **2 chopping boards**
- **2 sharp knives**
- **can opener**
- **1 colander**
- **1 saucepan**
- **1 tablespoon**
- **1 wooden spoon**
- **1 fork**

1. **Clear** your counter of clutter and **set out** all the equipment you need.
2. **Prepare** the stock according to the packet instructions.
3. **Quarter** the sausages.
4. **On a separate chopping board, with a new knife**, **chop** the onion and **core**, **deseed** and **chop** the red pepper. **Crush** (using the flat side of the knife) and **finely chop** the garlic.
5. **Drain** and **rinse** the mixed beans in a colander.
6. **Heat** the oil in a saucepan, **add** the onion, garlic and red pepper and **fry** over a **medium heat** for 2–3 minutes until they are beginning to soften.
7. **Add** the sausages and continue to **cook** for another 5 minutes until browned all over.
8. **Crush** half of the beans lightly with the back of a fork and **add** to the pan with the remaining beans, the tomatoes, stock and tomato purée. **Season** to taste with salt and pepper. Bring to the **boil** and **simmer** for 10 minutes. **Remove** the pan from the heat.
9. **Chop** the parsley, **scatter** it on top of the casserole and then **serve**.

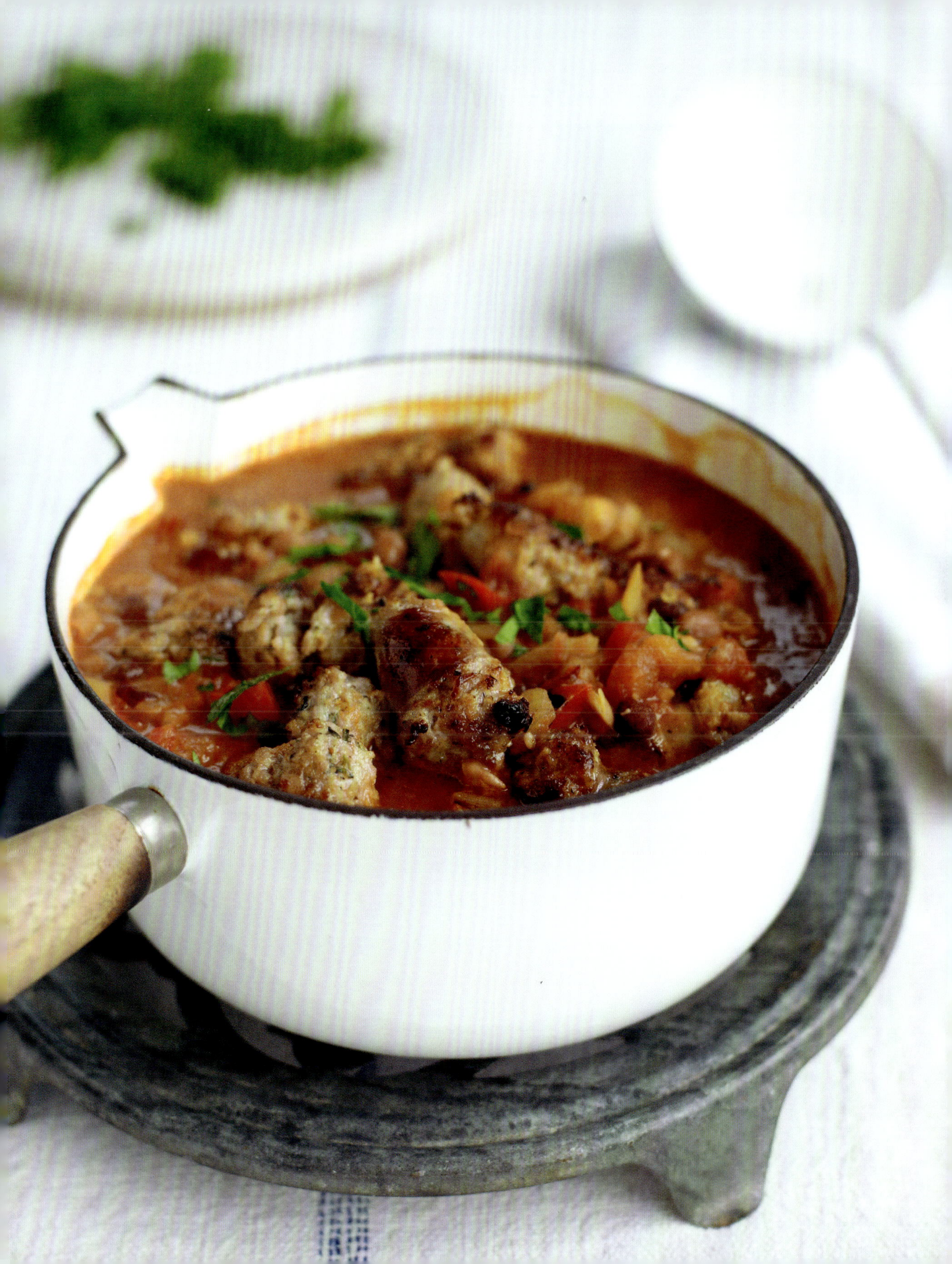

Serves 4 ▪ Preparation time: 10–15 minutes ▪ Cooking time: 15 minutes
Total time: 25–30 minutes

Tuna Enchiladas

Ingredients

- 2 ripe tomatoes
- 1 red onion
- ½ lime
- 300 g (10 oz) can tuna in spring water
- 150 g (5 oz) Cheddar cheese
- 8 chapattis
- salt and pepper
- fresh coriander, to garnish

Equipment

- kitchen scales
- 1 chopping board
- 1 sharp knife
- 1 bowl
- 1 mixing spoon
- 1 lemon juicer
- measuring spoons
- can opener
- 1 grater
- 1 spoon
- 1 ovenproof dish
- foil
- timer

1. **Clear** your counter of clutter and **set out** all the equipment you need.
2. **Preheat** the oven to **200°C (400°F), Gas Mark 6**.
3. **Chop** the tomatoes and **finely chop** the red onion. **Mix** them together in a bowl. **Juice** the lime and **add** 1 tablespoon of juice to the tomato salsa. **Season** well with salt and pepper.
4. **Drain** the tuna and **grate** the Cheddar.
5. **Spoon** some of the tomato salsa over each chapatti, **top** with the tuna and half the cheese. **Roll up** each chapatti and **arrange** them in an ovenproof dish. **Sprinkle** over the remaining cheese and any remaining tomato salsa.
6. **Cover** with foil and **cook** in the oven for 15 minutes until golden. **Set a timer** so you don't forget.
7. **Chop** the coriander and **sprinkle** over the enchiladas to garnish, then **serve**.

Serves 4 ▪ Preparation time: 5–10 minutes ▪ Cooking time: 10 minutes
Total time: 15–20 minutes

Sea Bass with Herb & Olive Couscous

Ingredients

- **350 ml (12 fl oz) hot vegetable stock**
- **1 ready-roasted red pepper from a jar**
- **handful of fresh basil**
- **handful of fresh parsley**
- **50 ml (2 fl oz) dry white wine**
- **300 g (10 oz) pearl couscous**
- **4 skinless sea bass fillets**
- **2 tablespoons extra virgin olive oil**
- **50 g (2 oz) pitted black olives**
- **salt and pepper**

Equipment

- **kitchen scales**
- **measuring jugs**
- **1 chopping board**
- **1 knife**
- **1 shallow, flameproof casserole dish with a lid**
- **1 wooden spoon**
- **measuring spoons**
- **1 spatula or fish slice**

1. **Clear** your counter of clutter and **set out** all the equipment you need.
2. **Prepare** the stock according to the packet instructions.
3. **Slice** the roasted red pepper. **Chop** the basil and parsley.
4. **Pour** the wine into a shallow, flameproof casserole dish and **boil** for 1 minute. **Add** the pearl couscous and stock and **stir** well, then **arrange** the sea bass fillets on top. **Cover** and leave to **cook** gently for 8 minutes until the fish and couscous are cooked through.
5. **Transfer** the sea bass to warmed plates, **stir** the oil, red pepper, olives, basil and parsley into the couscous. **Season** to taste with salt and pepper and **serve** with the fish.

Serves 2 ▪ Preparation time: 10–15 minutes ▪ Cooking time: 50 minutes
Total time: 1 hour–1 hour 5 minutes

Chilli con Carne

Ingredients

- 200 ml (7 fl oz) hot beef stock
- 1 red onion
- 3 garlic cloves
- 1 small red pepper
- 400 g (13 oz) can red kidney beans
- 2 tablespoons olive oil
- 250 g (8 oz) lean minced beef
- ½ teaspoon ground cumin
- 400 g (13 oz) can chopped tomatoes
- 1 tablespoon tomato purée
- 2 teaspoons mild chilli powder
- salt and pepper
- microwave brown rice, to serve

Equipment

- kitchen scales
- 1 measuring jug
- 1 chopping board
- 1 sharp knife
- can opener
- 1 colander
- 1 saucepan
- measuring spoons
- 1 wooden spoon
- timer

1. **Clear** your counter of clutter and **set out** all the equipment you need.
2. **Prepare** the stock according to the packet instructions.
3. **Finely chop** the red onion and garlic. **Core, deseed** and **dice** the red pepper.
4. **Drain** and **rinse** the kidney beans in a colander.
5. **Heat** the oil in a saucepan. **Add** the red onion and garlic and **cook** over a **medium-high heat** for 5 minutes or until beginning to soften. **Add** the minced beef and cumin and **cook** for a further 5–6 minutes or until browned all over. **Break up** the minced beef with a wooden spoon as it cooks.
6. **Stir** in the red pepper, tomatoes, tomato purée, chilli powder and stock and bring to the **boil**. **Reduce** the heat and **simmer** gently for 30 minutes. **Set a timer** every 10 minutes to remember to **stir**.
7. **Add** the kidney beans and **cook** for a further 5 minutes. **Season** to taste with salt and pepper.
8. **Microwave** the brown rice according to the packet instructions.
9. **Serve** the chilli with the brown rice.

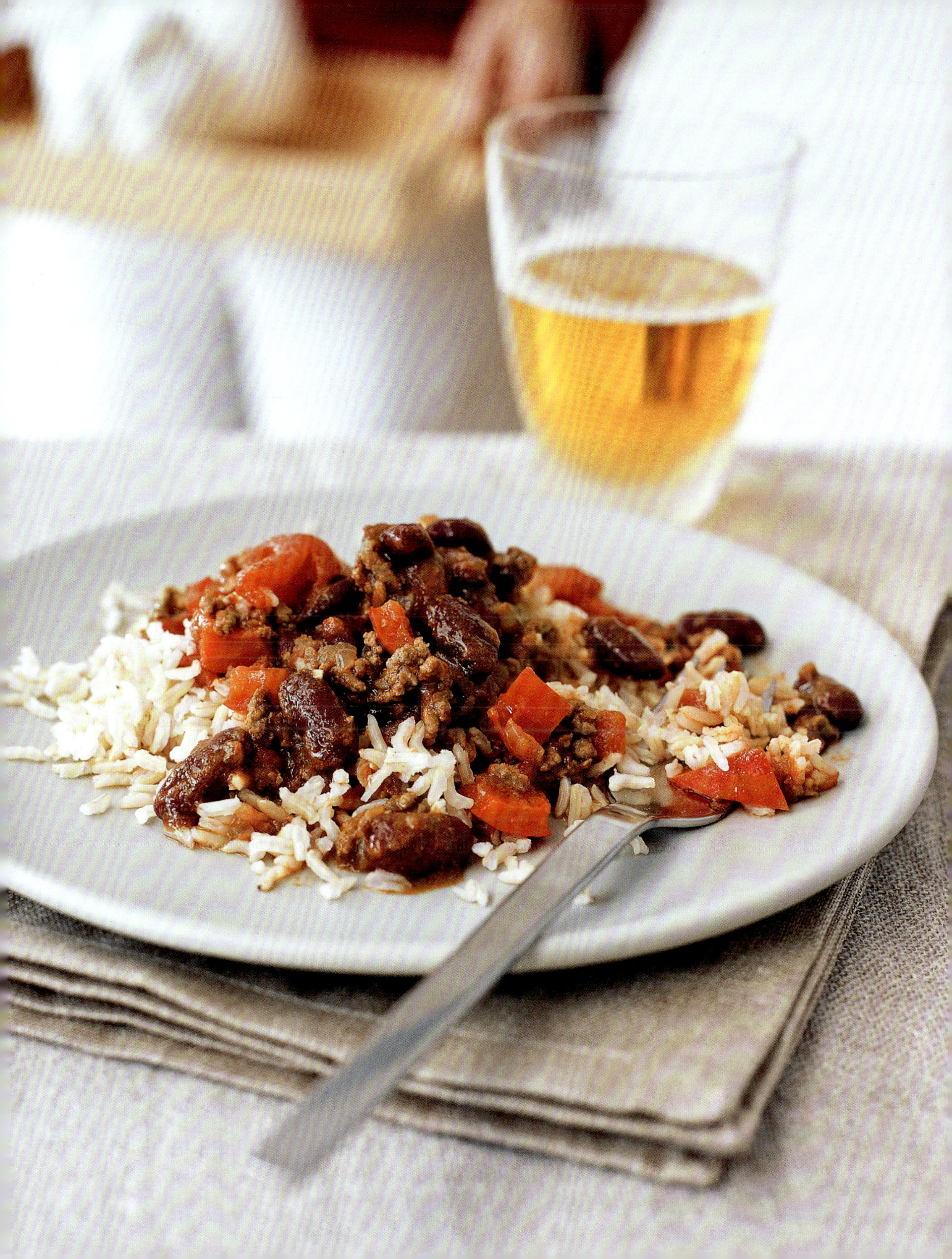

Serves 4 ▪ Preparation time: 10 minutes ▪ Cooking time: 20 minutes
Total time: 30 minutes

Rice with Salmon & Lemon Ponzu Dressing

Ingredients

- **2.5 cm (1 inch) piece of fresh root ginger**
- **1 red chilli**
- **1 lemon**
- **400 g (13 oz) jasmine rice**
- **1 litre (1¾ pints) water**
- **4 skinless salmon fillets**
- **75 g (3 oz) frozen shelled edamame beans**
- **4 tablespoons soy sauce**
- **1 tablespoon mirin**
- **salt**
- **1 spring onion, to garnish**

Equipment

- **kitchen scales**
- **1 measuring jug**
- **1 vegetable peeler**
- **1 chopping board**
- **1 sharp knife**
- **1 large, heavy-based casserole dish with a lid**
- **1 lemon juicer**
- **measuring spoons**
- **1 small bowl**
- **1 mixing spoon**

1. **Clear** your counter of clutter and **set out** all the equipment you need.
2. **Peel**, then **cut** the fresh root ginger into matchsticks. **Slice** the chilli, **halve** the lemon and **cut** one half into 4 slices.
3. **Put** the rice and measured water in a large, heavy-based casserole dish. **Add** a little salt and bring to the **boil**, then **reduce** the heat and **simmer**, uncovered, for 7 minutes until most of the water has boiled away.
4. **Place** the salmon fillets on top, **scatter** over the ginger and chilli and then **place** a lemon slice on each piece of fish. **Cover** and **cook** for a further 7 minutes until the fish is just cooked through.
5. **Scatter** over the edamame beans and **leave** to steam for 1–2 minutes until heated through.
6. **Juice** the remaining lemon half and **mix** 1 tablespoon of the juice together with the soy sauce and mirin. **Pour** over the fish.
7. **Slice** the spring onion and **scatter** over the salmon fillets to garnish, then **serve**.

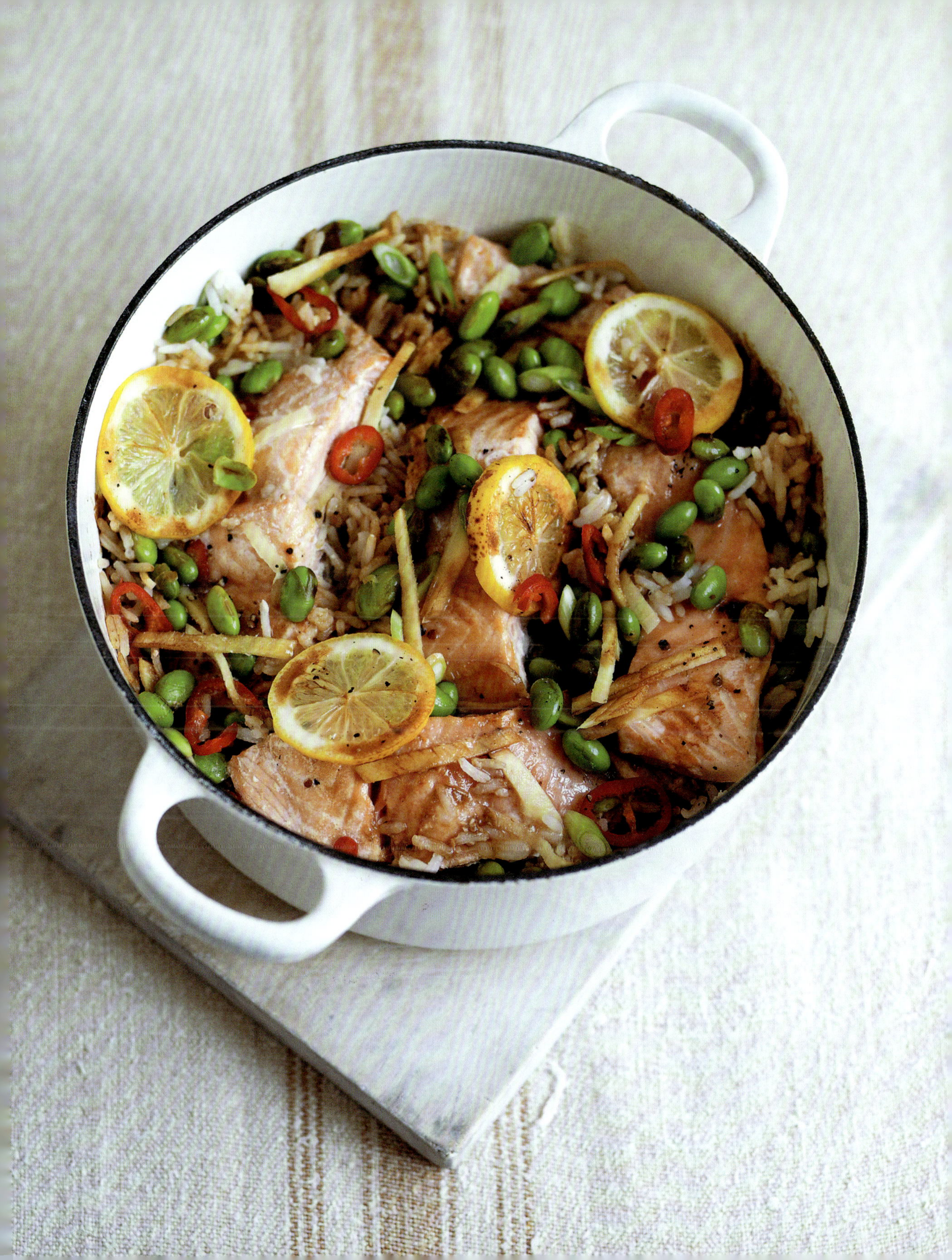

Serves 4 ▪ Preparation time: 10 minutes ▪ Cooking time: 10 minutes
Total time: 20 minutes

Chicken, Olive & Cumin Couscous

Ingredients

- **300 ml (½ pint) hot chicken stock**
- **2 ready-cooked chicken breasts**
- **½ lemon**
- **1 garlic clove**
- **400 g (13 oz) can chickpeas**
- **4 tablespoons olive oil**
- **1 tablespoon clear honey**
- **½ teaspoon ground cumin**
- **300 g (10 oz) couscous**
- **50 g (2 oz) pitted green olives**
- **handful of fresh coriander**
- **handful of fresh mint**
- **salt and pepper**

Equipment

- **kitchen scales**
- **1 measuring jug**
- **2 chopping boards**
- **2 sharp knives**
- **can opener**
- **1 colander**
- **1 saucepan**
- **1 wooden spoon**
- **measuring spoons**
- **1 fork**

1. **Clear** your counter of clutter and **set out** all the equipment you need.
2. **Prepare** the stock according to the packet instructions.
3. **Slice** the chicken breasts.
4. **On a separate chopping board, with a new knife, finely chop** the lemon (rind and flesh). **Crush** (using the flat side of the knife) and **finely chop** the garlic.
5. **Drain** and **rinse** the chickpeas in a colander.
6. **Heat** the oil and lemon in a saucepan and **cook** over a **gentle heat** for about 2 minutes until the lemon is soft.
7. **Stir** in the honey, cumin and garlic and **heat** through. **Stir** in the couscous, stock, chickpeas, olives and chicken.
8. **Remove** from the heat and **leave** for 5 minutes until the couscous is tender.
9. **Chop** the coriander and mint. **Fluff up** the couscous with a fork and **stir** in the coriander and mint. **Season** to taste with salt and pepper and **serve** immediately.

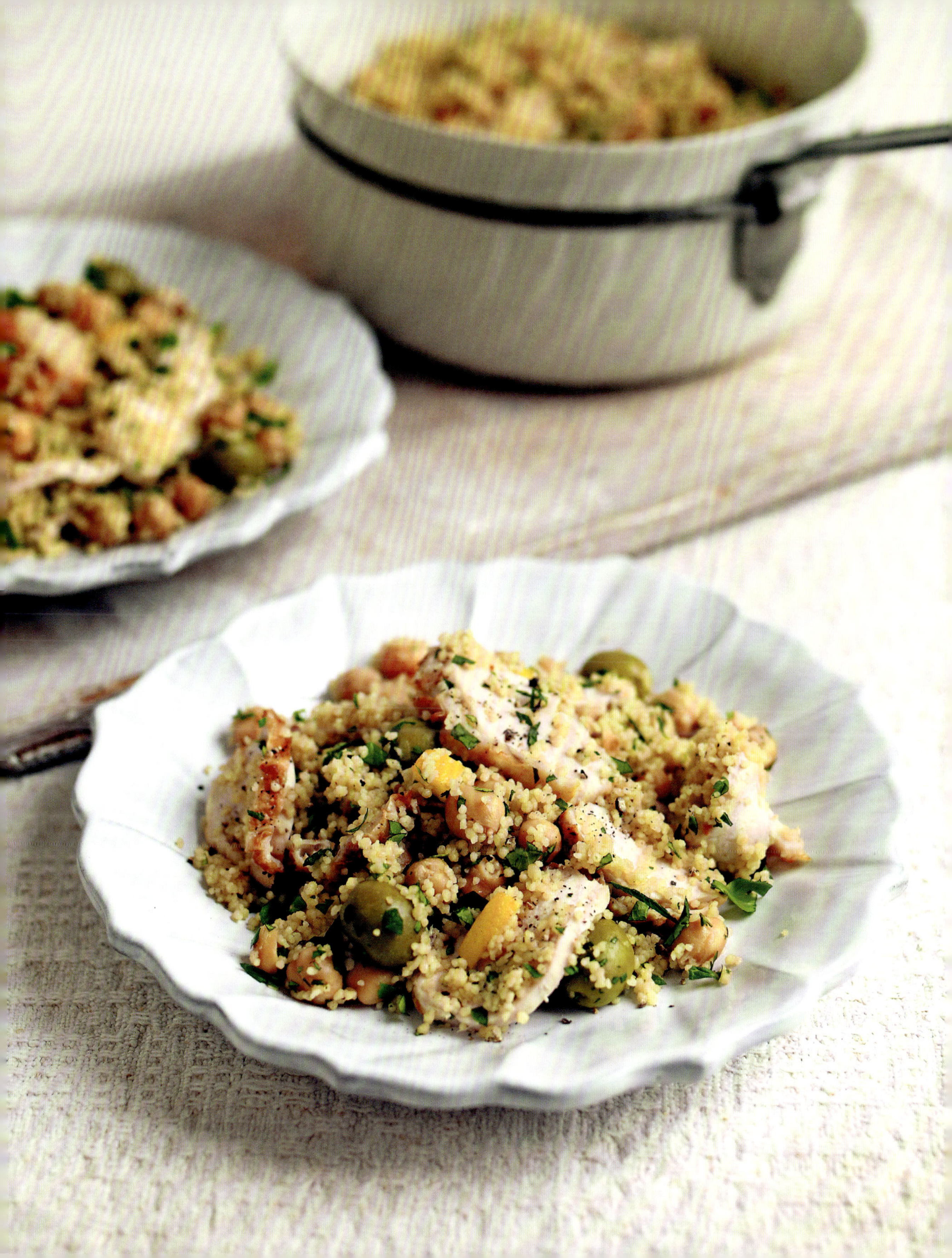

Serves 4 ▪ Preparation time: 5–10 minutes ▪ Cooking time: 25 minutes
Total time: 30–35 minutes

Chicken & Coconut Curry Rice

Ingredients

- **300 ml (½ pints) hot chicken stock**
- **1 onion**
- **1 red pepper**
- **1 garlic clove**
- **10 g (¼ oz) fresh root ginger**
- **1 tablespoon vegetable oil**
- **2 tablespoons Thai green curry paste**
- **325 g (11 oz) chicken mini-fillets**
- **250 g (8 oz) jasmine rice**
- **400 ml (14 fl oz) coconut milk**
- **handful of fresh basil**
- **1 lime**
- **salt and pepper**

Equipment

- **kitchen scales**
- **measuring jugs**
- **1 chopping board**
- **1 sharp knife**
- **1 vegetable peeler**
- **1 grater**
- **1 large, heavy-based saucepan with a lid**
- **measuring spoons**
- **1 wooden spoon**
- **can opener**

1. **Clear** your counter of clutter and **set out** all the equipment you need.
2. **Prepare** the stock according to the packet instructions.
3. **Finely chop** the onion and **core**, **deseed** and **thickly slice** the red pepper. **Crush** (using the flat side of the knife) and **finely chop** the garlic. **Peel** and **finely grate** the fresh root ginger.
4. **Heat** the oil in a large, heavy-based saucepan. Add the onion and **cook** over a **medium heat** for 5 minutes until softened. **Stir** in the garlic, ginger and curry paste and **cook** for a further 1 minute. **Add** the chicken and red pepper, followed by the rice, and **stir** well.
5. **Pour** in the coconut milk and stock and **season** to taste with salt and pepper. Bring to the **boil**, then **reduce** the heat and **simmer** for about 10 minutes until nearly all the liquid has boiled away, stirring once or twice.
6. **Turn the heat down** as low as it will go, **cover** the pan and **cook** for a further 5 minutes or until the rice is cooked through.
7. **Chop** the basil and **slice** the lime into wedges. **Sprinkle** the basil over the chicken and **serve** the rice hot with the lime wedges for squeezing.

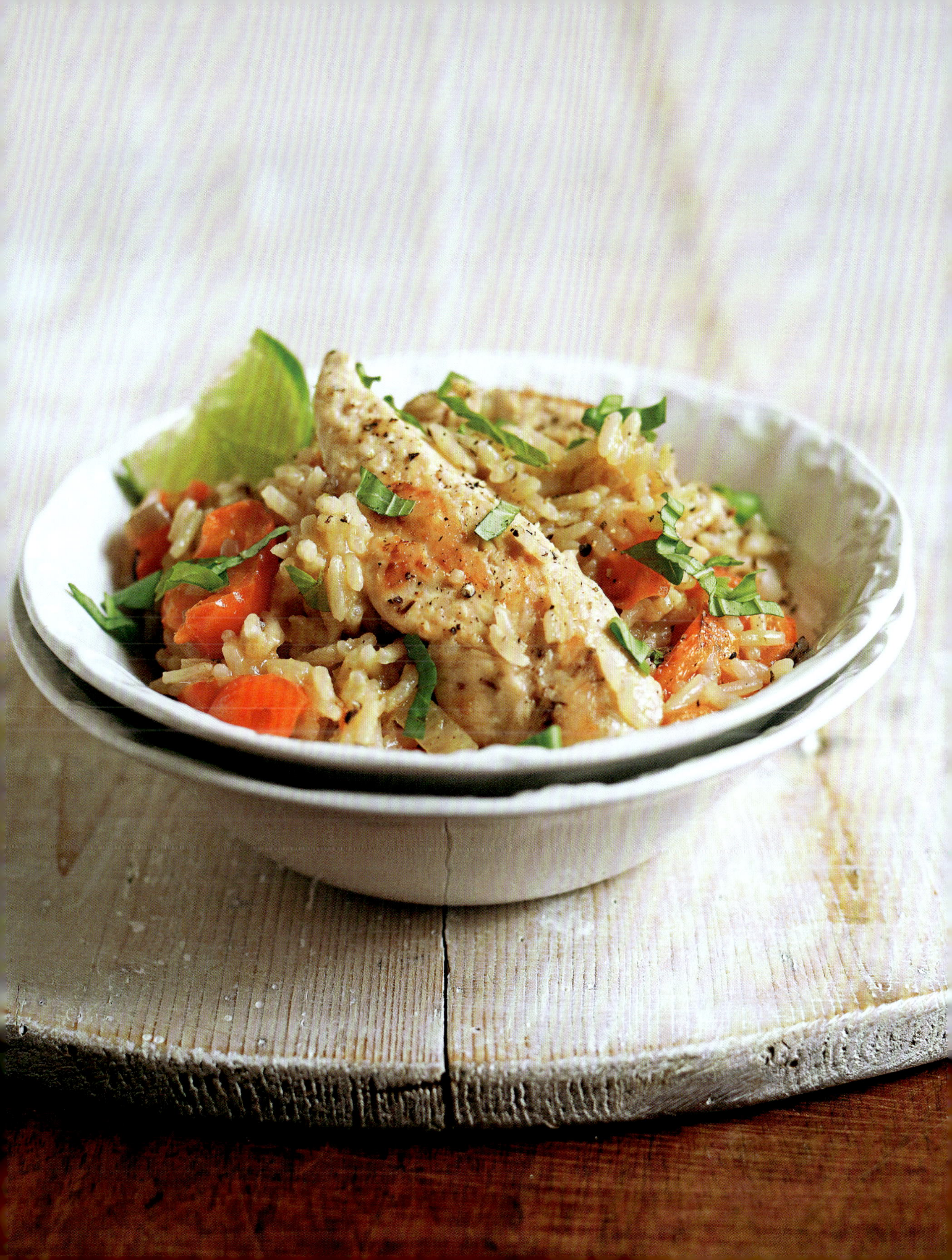

Serves 4 ▪ Preparation time: 10 minutes ▪ Cooking time: 20 minutes
Total time: 30 minutes

Salmon Tikka Masala

Ingredients

- 375 g (12 oz) salmon fillet
- 1 onion
- 1 red pepper
- 1 garlic clove
- 5 g (⅛ oz) fresh root ginger
- 2 tablespoons vegetable oil
- 3 tablespoons tikka masala paste
- 400 g (13 oz) can chopped tomatoes
- 75 ml (3 fl oz) single cream
- 75 ml (3 fl oz) natural yogurt
- salt and pepper
- small handful of fresh coriander, to garnish
- naan, to serve

Equipment

- kitchen scales
- measuring jugs
- 2 chopping boards
- 2 knives
- 1 vegetable peeler
- 1 grater
- 1 large saucepan
- measuring spoons
- 1 wooden spoon
- can opener

1. **Clear** your counter of clutter and **set out** all the equipment you need.
2. **Cut** the salmon into chunks.
3. **On a separate chopping board, with a new knife**, **slice** the onion and **core**, **deseed** and **slice** the red pepper. **Crush** (using the flat side of the knife) and **finely chop** the garlic. **Peel** and **grate** the fresh root ginger.
4. **Heat** the oil in a large saucepan. **Add** the onion, garlic and ginger and cook over a **medium heat** for 3 minutes until softened. **Add** the red pepper and **cook** for a further 2 minutes. **Stir** in the tikka masala paste followed by the tomatoes and bring to the **boil**. **Cook** for 5 minutes.
5. **Reduce** to a **simmer**, **add** the salmon and **season** with salt and pepper. **Cook** for 8 minutes or until cooked through. **Stir** through the cream and some of the yogurt, leaving a little to **drizzle** on top.
6. **Chop** the coriander and **scatter** it over the curry to garnish. **Serve** with naan on the side.

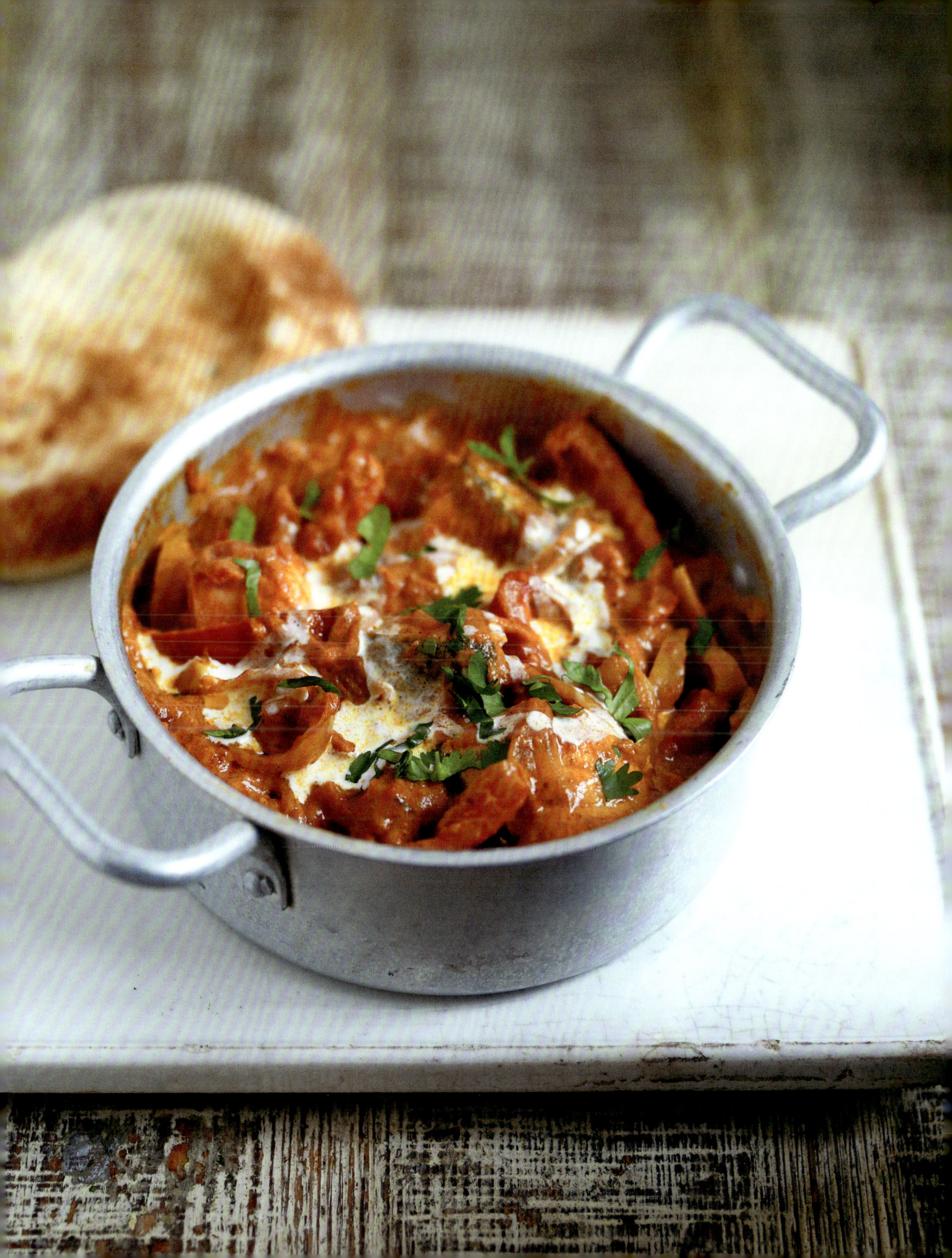

Sweet Treats

Makes 12 ▪ Preparation time: 15 minutes, plus cooling
Cooking time: 22 minutes ▪ Total time: 37 minutes

Wholemeal Raspberry Coconut Muffins

Ingredients

- **100 g (3½ oz) coconut oil**
- **150 g (5 oz) plain flour**
- **150 g (5 oz) plain wholemeal flour**
- **1 teaspoon baking powder**
- **2 eggs**
- **125 ml (4 fl oz) milk**
- **75 g (3 oz) light muscovado sugar**
- **225 g (7½ oz) fresh raspberries**
- **2 tablespoons desiccated coconut**

Equipment

- **kitchen scales**
- **12-hole muffin tin**
- **12 paper muffin cases**
- **1 small saucepan**
- **2 large bowls**
- **1 sieve**
- **measuring spoons**
- **1 whisk**
- **2 spoons**
- **timer**
- **1 wire rack**

1. **Clear** your counter of clutter and **set out** all the equipment you need.
2. **Preheat** the oven to **200°C (400°F), Gas Mark 6. Line** a 12-hole muffin tin with paper muffin cases.
3. **Put** the coconut oil in a small saucepan and **melt** over a low heat. **Set aside** to cool.
4. **Sift** the flours and baking powder into a large bowl.
5. **Beat** the eggs in a small bowl.
6. In a separate bowl, **whisk** together the melted coconut oil, eggs, milk and sugar, then **pour** into the dry ingredients and **mix** together until just combined – **do not over-mix.**
7. Gently **stir** in the raspberries, then **spoon** the mixture into the paper cases using 2 spoons and **sprinkle** with the desiccated coconut.
8. **Bake** in the oven for 20 minutes or until risen, golden and firm to the touch. **Set a timer** so you don't forget.
9. **Transfer** to a wire rack to cool, then **serve.** Leftover muffins can be stored in an airtight container for up to 3 days.

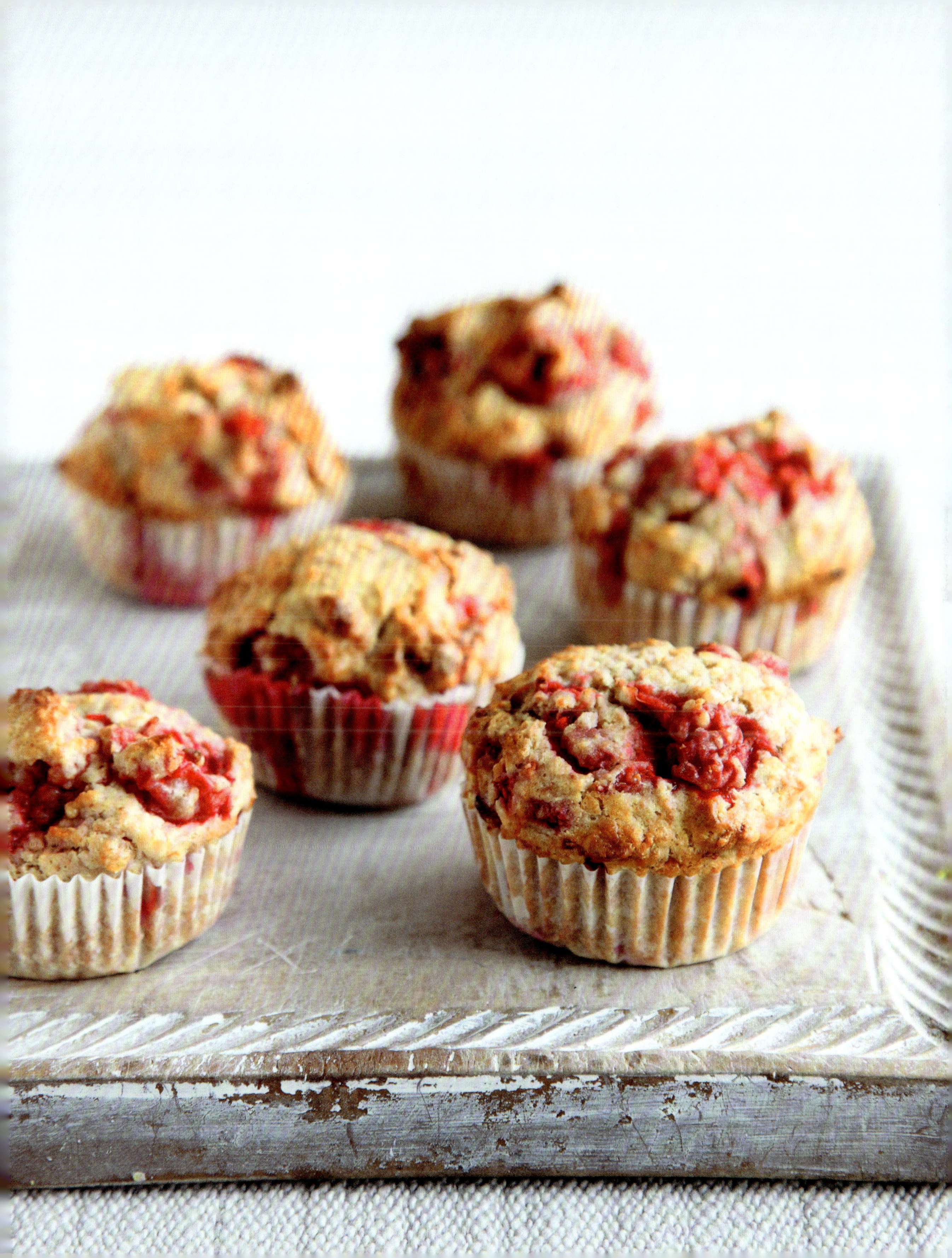

Makes 12 ▪ Preparation time: 10–15 minutes ▪ Cooking time: 18 minutes
Total time: 28–33 minutes

Lemon Yogurt Cupcakes

Ingredients

- 2 eggs
- ½ lemon
- 100 ml (3½ fl oz) groundnut oil
- 125 ml (4 fl oz) natural yogurt
- 100 g (3½ oz) golden caster sugar
- 150 g (5 oz) plain flour
- 50 g (2 oz) ground almonds
- 1 teaspoon baking powder
- ½ teaspoon bicarbonate of soda
- pinch of salt

Equipment

- kitchen scales
- measuring jugs
- 12-hole cupcake or muffin tin
- 12 small silicone or paper cupcake cases
- 1 small bowl
- 1 fork
- 1 grater
- 1 large bowl
- measuring spoons
- 1 wooden spoon
- 2 spoons
- timer
- 1 wire rack

1. **Clear** your counter of clutter and **set out** all the equipment you need.
2. **Preheat** the oven to **180°C (350°F), Gas Mark 4**. **Line** a 12-hole cupcake or muffin tin with small silicone or paper cupcake cases.
3. **Lightly beat** the eggs in a small bowl with a fork. **Finely grate** the lemon rind.
4. **Put** all the ingredients in a large bowl and **beat** together until smooth, then **spoon** the batter into the cake cases using 2 spoons. **Bake** the cakes in the oven for 18 minutes or until risen, golden and firm to the touch. **Set a timer** so you don't forget.
5. **Remove** from the oven and **transfer** the cupcakes to a wire rack. **Serve** warm or cold. Leftover muffins can be stored in an airtight container for up to 3 days.

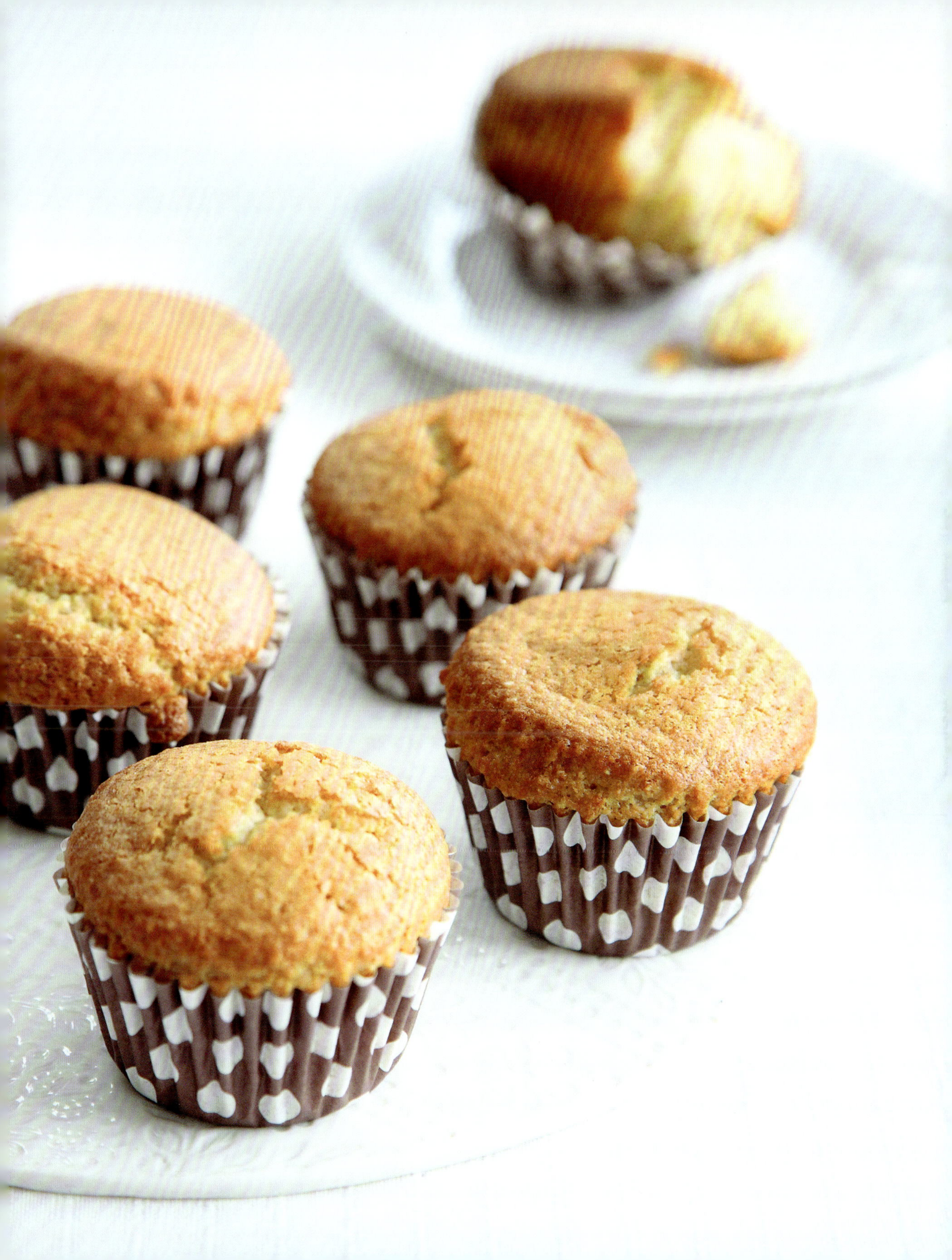

Makes 12 • Preparation time: 10–15 minutes • Cooking time: 22 minutes
Total time: 32–37 minutes

Banana, Oat & Almond Muffins

Ingredients

- **1 large banana**
- **75 g (3 oz) slightly salted butter, plus extra to serve**
- **1 egg**
- **2 tablespoons clear honey, plus extra to serve**
- **150 ml (¼ pint) full-fat milk**
- **175 g (6 oz) self-raising flour**
- **75 g (3 oz) porridge oats**
- **1 teaspoon baking powder**
- **25 g (1 oz) ground almonds**
- **25 g (1 oz) flaked almonds**

Equipment

- **kitchen scales**
- **1 measuring jug**
- **12-hole muffin tin**
- **12 paper muffin cases**
- **1 chopping board**
- **1 knife**
- **1 small saucepan**
- **1 jug**
- **1 fork**
- **measuring spoons**
- **1 large bowl**
- **1 mixing spoon**
- **2 spoons**
- **timer**

1. **Clear** your counter of clutter and **set out** all the equipment you need.
2. **Preheat** the oven to **200°C (400°F), Gas Mark 6. Line** a 12-hole muffin tin with paper muffin cases.
3. **Peel** and **roughly chop** the banana.
4. **Melt** the butter in a small saucepan.
5. **Beat** the egg in a jug, then **add** the melted butter, honey and milk and **mix** together.
6. **Put** the banana, flour, oats, baking powder and ground and flaked almonds in a large bowl.
7. **Pour** in the milk mixture and quickly **mix** together all the ingredients to give a fairly lumpy mixture (this will give the muffins their lightness).
8. **Spoon** the batter into the paper cases using 2 spoons. **Bake** in the oven for about 20 minutes until golden and firm to the touch. **Set a timer** so you don't forget.
9. **Serve** warm with extra butter and honey. Leftover muffins can be stored in an airtight container for up to 3 days.

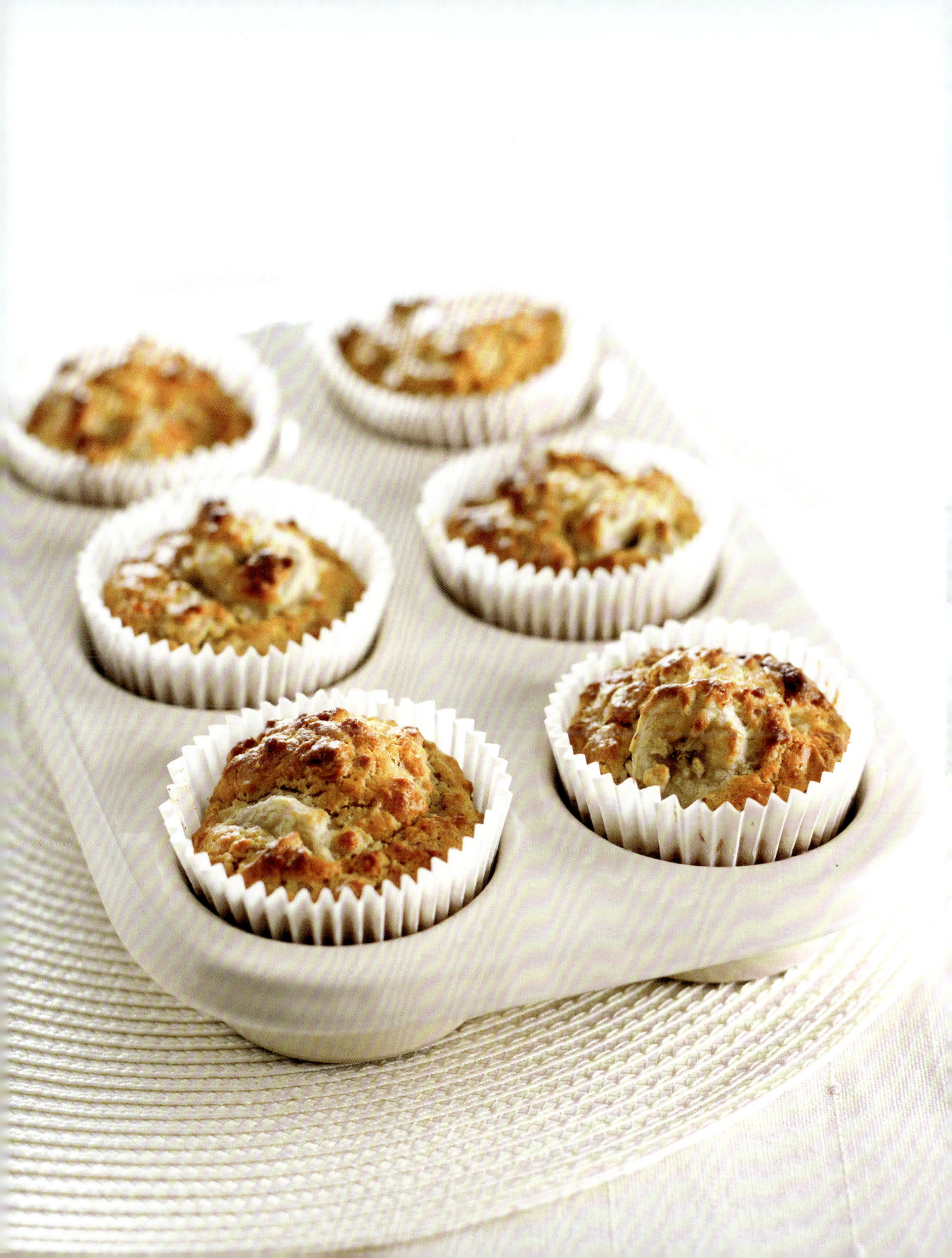

Cuts into 16 ▪ Preparation time: 20 minutes ▪ Cooking time: 40–45 minutes
Total time: 1 hour–1 hour 5 minutes

Squidgy Apple Cake

Ingredients

- **250 g (8 oz) slightly salted butter, softened, plus extra for greasing**
- **250 g (8 oz) golden caster sugar, plus extra for sprinkling**
- **2 teaspoons mixed spice**
- **4 eggs**
- **300 g (10 oz) self-raising flour**
- **1 teaspoon baking powder**
- **4 tart dessert apples**

Equipment

- **kitchen scales**
- **32 × 22 cm (12½ × 8½ inch) shallow baking tin**
- **nonstick baking paper**
- **1 large bowl**
- **measuring spoons**
- **1 hand-held electric whisk**
- **1 vegetable peeler**
- **1 grater**
- **1 mixing spoon**
- **1 rubber spatula**
- **timer**
- **1 skewer**
- **1 sharp knife**

1. **Clear** your counter of clutter and **set out** all the equipment you need.
2. **Preheat** the oven to **180°C (350°F), Gas Mark 4. Grease** and **line** a 32 × 22 cm (12½ × 8½ inch) shallow baking tin with nonstick baking paper.
3. **Peel**, **core** and **coarsely grate** 3 of the apples.
4. **Beat** together the butter, sugar, mixed spice, eggs, half of the flour and the baking powder in a large bowl until pale and creamy. **Add** the grated apple to the bowl, then **stir** gently to combine. **Stir** in the remaining flour.
5. **Spoon** the mixture into the prepared tin and **level** the surface. **Peel**, **core** and **grate** the remaining apple evenly over the surface.
6. **Bake** in the oven for 40–45 minutes until golden, just firm to the touch and a skewer inserted into the centre comes out clean. **Set a timer** so you don't forget.
7. **Remove** from the oven, **sprinkle** with extra caster sugar and **leave to cool** in the tin. **Turn out**, **peel off** the lining paper and **cut** into 16 squares, then **serve**, warm or cold. Leftovers can be stored in an airtight container for 3 days.

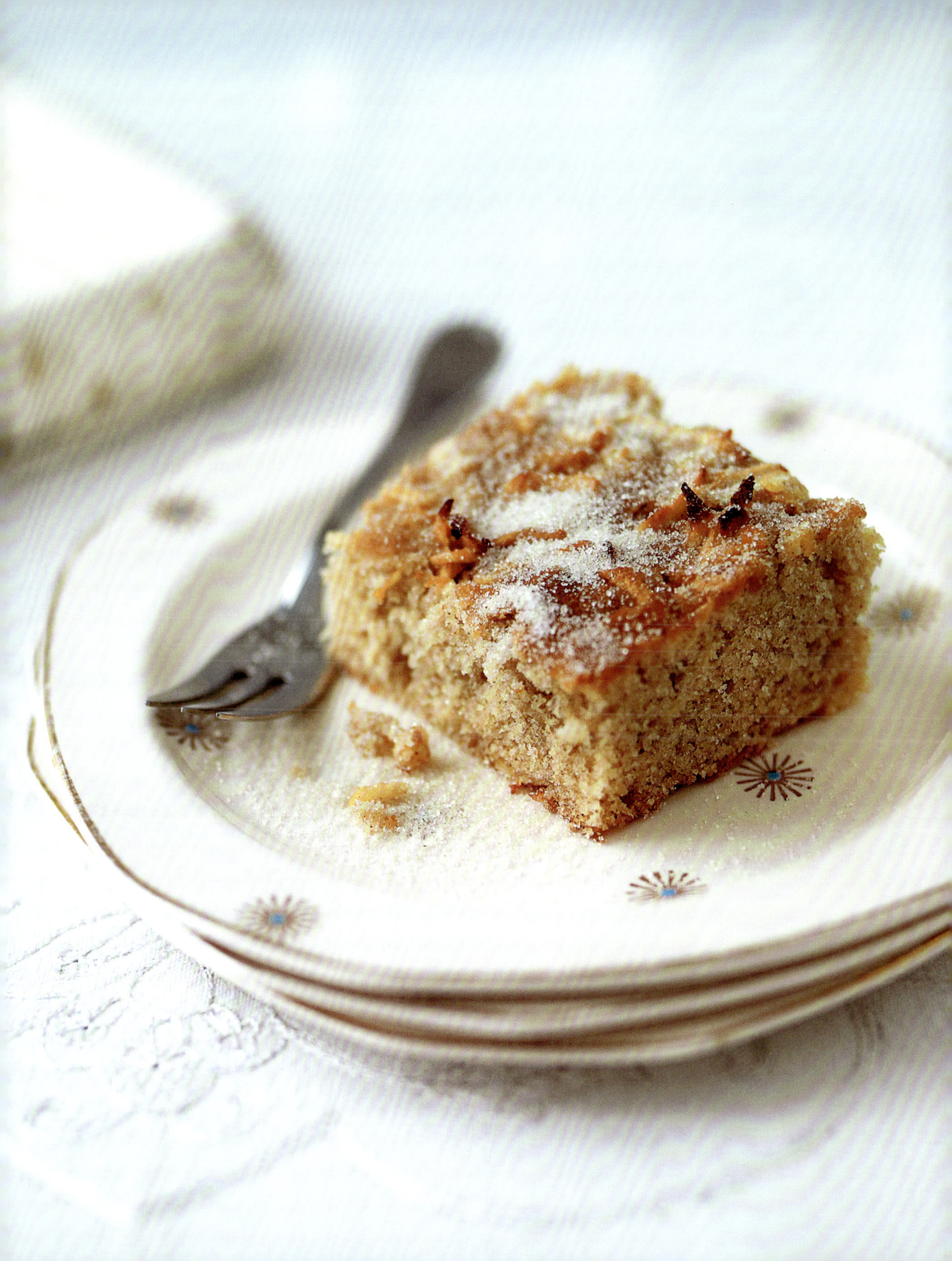

Serves 4 ▪ Preparation time: 5 minutes, plus cooling
Cooking time: 2–3 minutes ▪ Total time: 7–8 minutes

Blackberry Brûlées

Ingredients

- **225 g (7½ oz) fresh blackberries**
- **2 tablespoons apple juice**
- **2–3 teaspoons caster sugar, to taste**
- **8 tablespoons Greek yogurt**
- **2 tablespoons soft dark brown sugar**

Equipment

- **kitchen scales**
- **measuring spoons**
- **1 saucepan**
- **2 spoons**
- **4 ramekins**

1. **Clear** your counter of clutter and **set out** all the equipment you need.
2. **Place** the blackberries, apple juice and caster sugar in a saucepan and **simmer** for 2–3 minutes. **Spoon** into 4 ramekins and **leave to cool**.
3. **Spoon** over the yogurt, then **sprinkle** with the brown sugar.
4. **Cover** and **chill** in the refrigerator until required.

Serves 10 ▪ Preparation time: 25 minutes ▪ Cooking time: 1 hour 10 minutes–1 hour 15 minutes ▪ Total time: 1 hour 35 minutes–1 hour 40 minutes

Banana, Date & Walnut Loaf

Ingredients

- vegetable oil, for greasing
- ½ lemon
- 400 g (13 oz) bananas
- 125 g (4 oz) butter
- 2 eggs
- 300 g (10 oz) self-raising flour
- 1 teaspoon baking powder
- 125 g (4 oz) caster sugar
- 175 g (6 oz) ready-chopped dried dates
- 50 g (2 oz) walnut pieces
- walnut halves
- banana chips

Equipment

- kitchen scales
- 1 kg (2 lb) loaf tin
- greaseproof paper
- 1 fork
- 1 lemon juicer
- measuring spoons
- 1 small bowl
- 1 small saucepan
- 1 jug
- 1 mixing bowl
- 1 mixing spoon
- 1 skewer
- timer
- 1 wire rack

1. **Clear** your counter of clutter and **set out** all the equipment you need.
2. **Preheat** the oven to **160°C (325°F), Gas Mark 3**. **Grease** a 1 kg (2 lb) loaf tin with oil and **line** its base and 2 long sides with oiled greaseproof paper.
3. **Juice** the lemon and put 1 tablespoon of juice in a small bowl. **Peel** then **mash** the bananas with the lemon juice.
4. **Put** the butter in a small saucepan and **melt** over a **low heat**. **Beat** the eggs in a jug.
5. **Put** the flour, baking powder and sugar in a mixing bowl. **Add** the mashed bananas, melted butter and eggs and **mix** together. **Stir** in the dates and walnut pieces, then **spoon** into the prepared tin. **Level** the surface and **decorate** the top with walnut halves and banana chips.
6. **Bake** in the centre of the oven for 1 hour 10 minutes–1 hour 15 minutes until well risen, the top has cracked and a skewer inserted into the centre comes out clean. **Set a timer** to check after 1 hour. Then **set a timer** every 5 minutes to avoid burning.
7. **Leave to cool** in the tin for 10 minutes, then **loosen** the edges, **turn out** on to a wire rack and **peel off** the lining paper. **Leave to cool** completely. Store in an airtight container for up to 5 days.

Makes 12 bars • Preparation time: 20 minutes • Cooking time: 50–60 minutes
Total time: 1 hour 10 minutes–1 hour 20 minutes

Blueberry & Oat Bars

Ingredients

- 175 g (6 oz) slightly salted butter, chilled, plus extra for greasing
- 100 g (3½ oz) plain wholemeal flour
- 75 g (3 oz) self-raising flour
- ½ teaspoon ground cinnamon
- 175 g (6 oz) porridge oats
- 150 g (5 oz) light muscovado sugar
- 200 g (7 oz) fresh blueberries
- vanilla sugar, for sprinkling

Equipment

- kitchen scales
- 28 × 18 cm (11 × 7 inch) shallow baking tin
- 1 bowl or food processor
- 1 chopping board
- 1 sharp knife
- measuring spoons
- 1 mixing spoon
- timer

1. **Clear** your counter of clutter and **set out** all the equipment you need.
2. **Preheat** the oven to **180°C (350°F), Gas Mark 4**. **Grease** a 28 × 18 cm (11 × 7 inch) shallow baking tin with butter.
3. **Put** the flours in a bowl or food processor. **Dice** and **add** the butter and **rub** in with the fingertips or **process** until the mixture resembles breadcrumbs. **Add** the cinnamon, oats and muscovado sugar and **stir** in or **process** briefly until the mixture makes coarse crumbs and starts to cling together.
4. **Tip** about half the crumble mixture into the prepared tin and **spread** in an even layer. **Pack down** with the back of a spoon to make a firm base. **Scatter** with the blueberries and **sprinkle** with the remaining crumble mixture.
5. **Bake** in the oven for about 50–60 minutes until the crumble is deep golden. **Set a timer** for 50 minutes to check. **Leave to cool** in the tin, then **sprinkle** with vanilla sugar and **cut** into bars to **serve**. Store in an airtight container for up to 3 days.

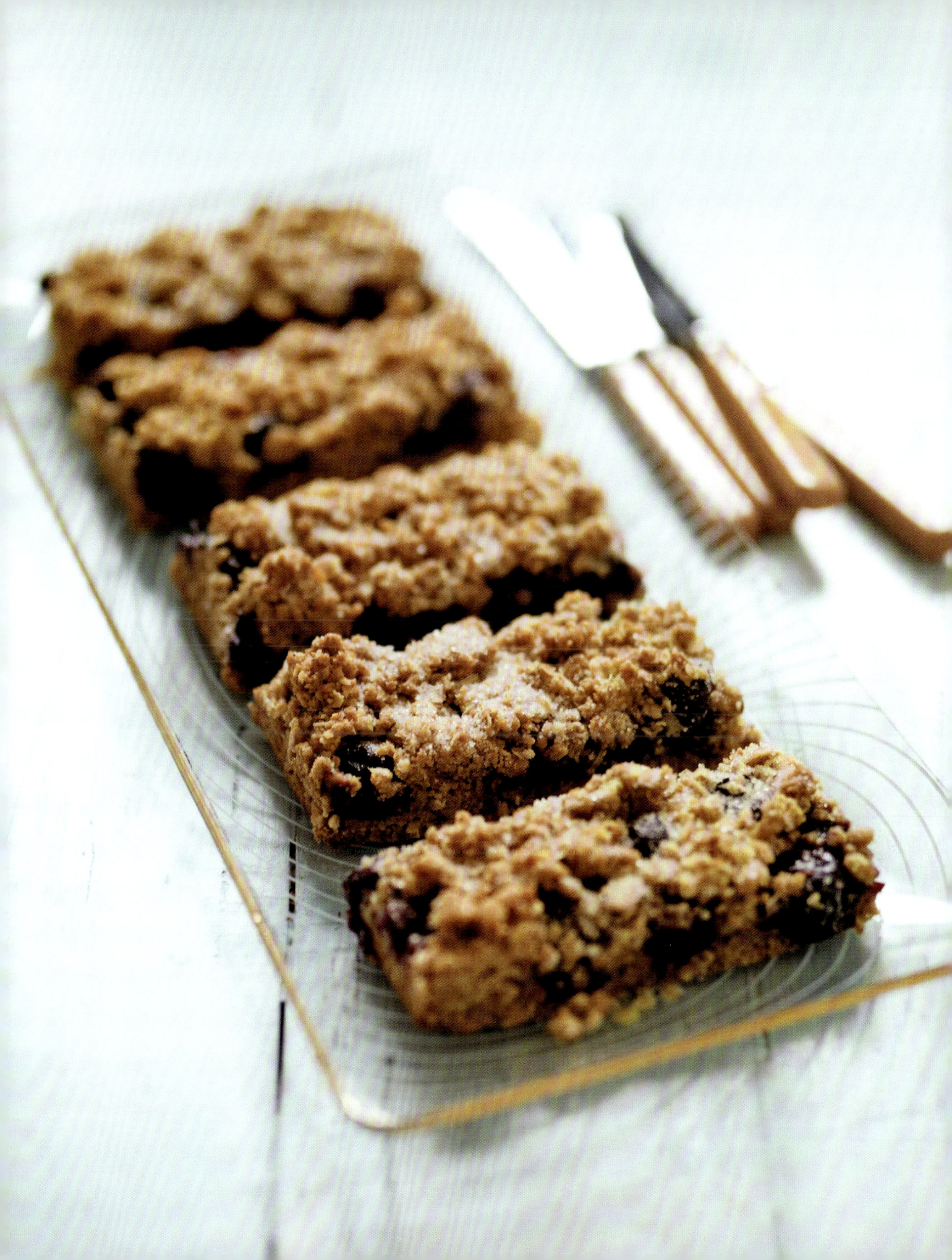

Serves 4 ▪ Preparation time: 10–15 minutes ▪ Cooking time: 1–2 minutes
Total time: 11–17 minutes

Date & Pistachio Bites

Ingredients

- **225 g (7½ oz) shelled pistachio nuts**
- **225 g (7½ oz) ready-to-eat pitted dates**
- **1 tablespoon orange blossom water**
- **1 teaspoon ground cinnamon**
- **1 tablespoon clear honey**
- **50 g (2 oz) desiccated coconut**

Equipment

- **kitchen scales**
- **1 heavy-based frying pan**
- **1 wooden spoon**
- **1 chopping board**
- **1 sharp knife**
- **1 food processor**
- **1 rubber spatula**
- **1 bowl**
- **measuring spoons**
- **1 plate**

1. **Clear** your counter of clutter and **set out** all the equipment you need.
2. Gently **heat** the pistachios in a dry heavy-based frying pan over a **medium heat** for 1–2 minutes, **stirring**, until they begin to colour and emit a nutty aroma. **Remove** from the heat.
3. **Chop** the dates and put into a food processor with the pistachios and **blend** to a thick paste.
4. **Transfer** the paste to a bowl and **knead** in the orange blossom water, cinnamon and honey. **Roll** about 16 small pieces of the mixture into bite-sized balls.
5. **Sprinkle** the desiccated coconut onto a plate. **Roll** the truffles in the coconut until evenly coated. **Serve** with coffee or tea. Store in an airtight container for up to 5 days.

Makes 24 ▪ Preparation time: 15 minutes ▪ Cooking time: 10–15 minutes
Total time: 25–30 minutes

Apricot, Fig & Mixed Seed Bites

Ingredients

- **50 g (2 oz) soft dried apricots**
- **50 g (2 oz) soft dried figs**
- **150 g (5 oz) butter**
- **75 g (3 oz) soft light brown sugar**
- **1 egg**
- **2 tablespoons water**
- **75 g (3 oz) plain wholemeal flour**
- **½ teaspoon bicarbonate of soda**
- **100 g (3½ oz) rolled oats**
- **50 g (2 oz) mixed seeds, such as pumpkin, sunflower and sesame**

Equipment

- **kitchen scales**
- **2 baking sheets**
- **greaseproof paper**
- **1 chopping board**
- **1 sharp knife**
- **1 bowl**
- **1 hand-held electric whisk**
- **measuring spoons**
- **1 sieve**
- **1 mixing spoon**
- **timer**
- **1 wire rack**

1. **Clear** your counter of clutter and **set out** all the equipment you need.
2. **Preheat** the oven to **180°C (350°F), Gas Mark 4**. **Line** 2 baking sheets with greaseproof paper.
3. **Chop** the apricots and figs.
4. **Beat** together the butter and sugar in a bowl using a hand-held electric whisk until light and fluffy, then **beat** in the egg and measured water.
5. **Sift** together the flour and bicarbonate of soda into the bowl, **adding** any bran in the sieve. **Add** the oats, apricots, figs and mixed seeds, then **fold** all the ingredients into the butter and sugar mixture.
6. **Place** walnut-sized pieces of the mixture on the prepared baking sheets (12 on each baking sheet, spacing them apart) and **flatten** them slightly with the back of a spoon.
7. **Bake** in the oven for 10–15 minutes until golden. **Set a timer** so you don't forget.
8. **Transfer** to a wire rack to cool. Store in an airtight container for up to 5 days.

Makes 15 ▪ Preparation time: 20 minutes ▪ Cooking time: 35 minutes
Total time: 50–55 minutes

Rich Chocolate Brownies

Ingredients

- 175 g (6 oz) slightly salted butter, plus extra for greasing
- 400 g (13 oz) plain dark chocolate
- 3 eggs
- 225 g (7½ oz) light muscovado sugar
- 100 g (3½ oz) self-raising flour
- crème fraîche, to serve (optional)

Equipment

- kitchen scales
- 28 × 18 cm (11 × 7 inch) shallow baking tin
- 1 chopping board
- 1 sharp knife
- 1 heatproof bowl
- 1 saucepan
- 1 mixing bowl
- 1 hand-held electric whisk
- 1 mixing spoon
- 1 rubber spatula
- timer

1. **Clear** your counter of clutter and **set out** all the equipment you need.
2. **Preheat** the oven to **190°C (375°F), Gas Mark 5**. **Grease** and **line** a 28 × 18 cm (11 × 7 inch) shallow baking tin.
3. **Chop** 150 g (5 oz) of the chocolate into 5 mm (¼ inch) pieces. **Break** the remaining chocolate into pieces and **put** in a heatproof bowl. **Dice** the butter, then add to the bowl with the chocolate. **Melt** over a saucepan of gently simmering water (don't let the base of the bowl touch the water).
4. **Beat** the eggs and sugar in a separate mixing bowl until light and foamy. **Stir** in the melted chocolate mixture. **Tip** in the flour and chopped chocolate and **mix** together until just combined.
5. **Spoon** the mixture into the prepared tin and **level** the surface. **Bake** in the oven for about 30 minutes or until a crust has formed but the mixture feels quite soft underneath. **Set a timer** for 30 minutes to remember to check, and then every 2 minutes after that until the brownies are done.
6. **Leave to cool** in the tin, then **transfer** to a board and **cut** into 15 small squares. **Serve** with crème fraîche, if liked. Store in an airtight container for up to 3 days.

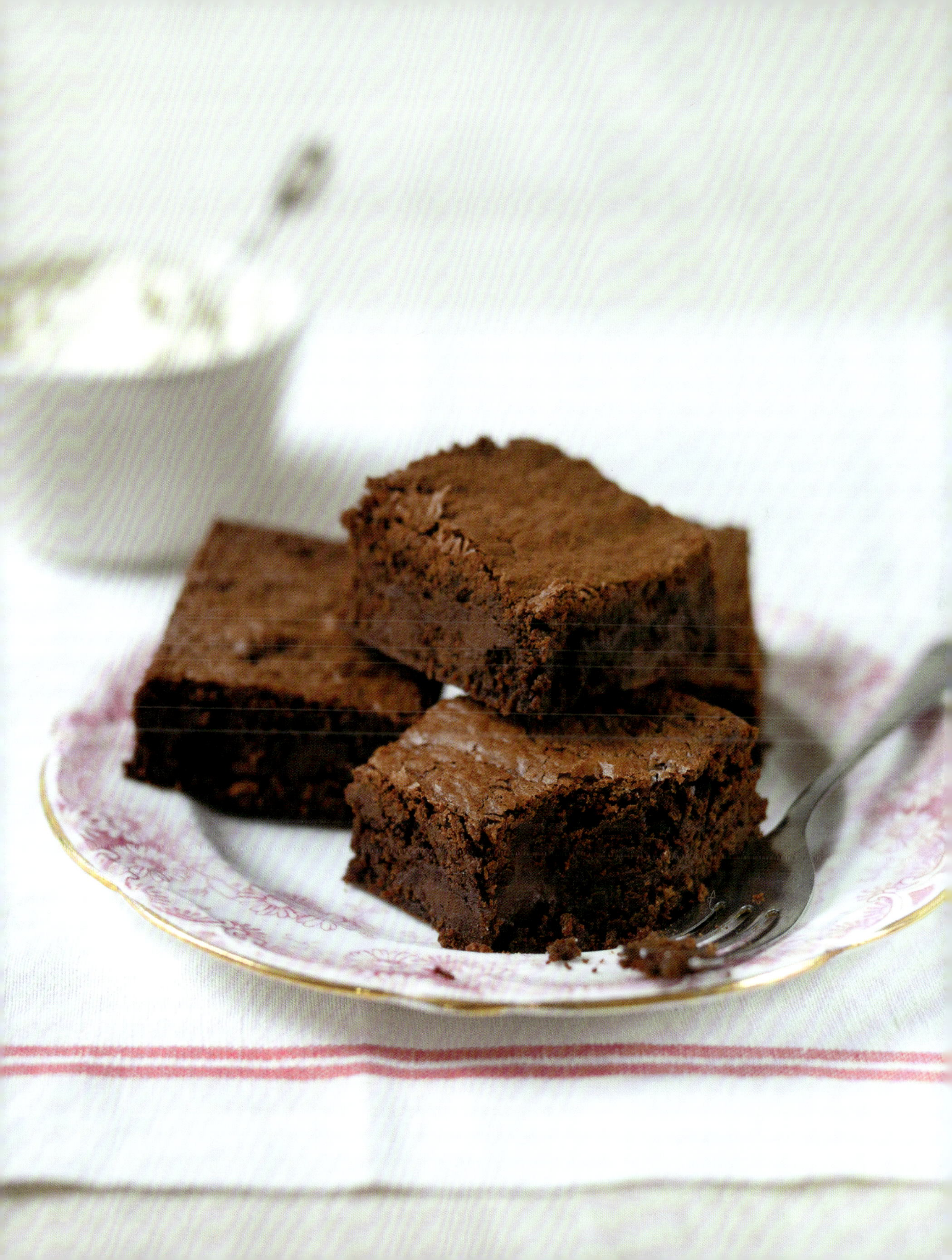

Serves 4 ▪ Preparation time: 10 minutes ▪ Cooking time: 4–6 minutes
Total time: 14–16 minutes

Griddled Peaches & Apricots with Honey Yogurt

Ingredients

- 200 ml (7 fl oz) Greek yogurt
- 2 tablespoons clear honey
- 3 fresh peaches
- 4 fresh apricots
- 2 tablespoons vanilla sugar

Equipment

- measuring jug
- 1 bowl
- measuring spoons
- 1 chopping board
- 1 sharp knife
- 1 large bowl
- 1 mixing bowl
- 1 griddle pan
- 1 set of tongs

1. **Clear** your counter of clutter and **set out** all the equipment you need.
2. **Place** the yogurt in a bowl and **pour** over the honey. **Stir** to create a rippled effect. **Set aside.**
3. **Halve**, **stone** and **quarter** the peaches. **Halve** and **stone** the apricots.
4. **Place** the vanilla sugar in a large bowl, then **add** the fruit and **toss** gently to coat.
5. **Preheat** a griddle pan until hot, then **add** the peaches, cut side down, and **griddle** over a **medium heat** for 2–3 minutes until caramelized, then **add** the apricots, cut side down. **Turn over** the peaches to the other cut side and **cook** for a further 2–3 minutes or until the apricots and peaches are soft.
6. **Serve** the warmed griddled fruit with the honey yogurt.

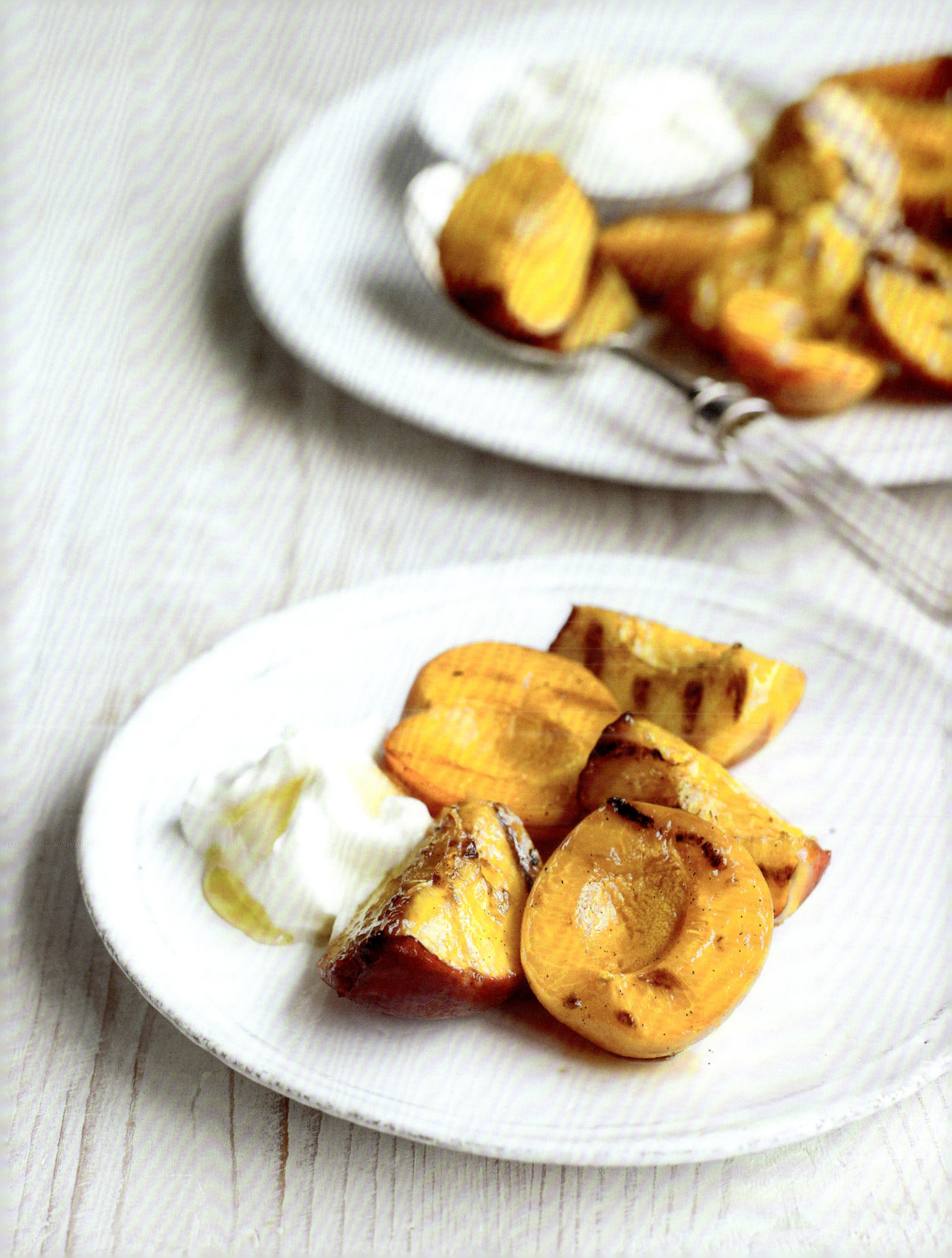

Serves 6–8 ▪ Preparation time: 15 minutes ▪ Cooking time: None
Total time: 15 minutes

Mixed Fruit Salad

Ingredients

- ¼ watermelon
- ½ galia melon
- 1 ripe mango
- 2 green dessert apples
- 2 bananas
- 3 kiwifruit
- 200 g (7 oz) fresh strawberries
- 150 g (5 oz) fresh blueberries

Equipment

- kitchen scales
- 1 chopping board
- 1 vegetable peeler
- 1 sharp knife
- 1 large bowl
- 1 mixing spoon

1. **Clear** your counter of clutter and **set out** all the equipment you need.
2. **Peel** and **deseed** both the melons and **cut** the flesh into 2–3 cm (1 inch) chunks. **Put** them in a large bowl. **Peel**, **stone** and **dice** the mango, **core** and **dice** the apples and **peel** and **slice** the bananas. **Add** to the bowl with the melon.
3. **Peel** the kiwifruit and **cut** the flesh into rounds, **add** to the bowl along with the berries and **mix** the fruit together carefully. **Serve**.

Serves 4 • Preparation time: 10 minutes, plus optional freezing
Cooking time: None • Total time: 10 minutes

Instant Raspberry Sorbet

Ingredients

- 300 g (10 oz) frozen raspberries
- 2 tablespoons caster sugar
- 2 tablespoons water
- 1 tablespoon crème de framboise (raspberry liqueur) (optional)
- fresh raspberries, to serve

Equipment

- kitchen scales
- 1 food processor
- 1 tablespoon
- 1 ice cream scoop

1. **Clear** your counter of clutter and **set out** all the equipment you need.
2. **Place** the frozen raspberries, sugar, measured water and crème de framboise, if using, in a food processor. **Blitz** for 2–3 minutes until all the ingredients are blended and come together.
3. **Serve** scoops of the sorbet immediately into bowls with some fresh raspberries, or place in a freezerproof container, cover and freeze for up to 1 month until ready to use.

Serves 4 ▪ Preparation time: 15 minutes, plus freezing ▪ Cooking time: None
Total time: 15 minutes

Frozen Fruity Yogurt

Ingredients

- **3 fresh nectarines**
- **300 g (10 oz) fresh or frozen raspberries**
- **2 tablespoons icing sugar**
- **600 ml (1 pint) Greek yogurt**

Equipment

- **kitchen scales**
- **1 measuring jug**
- **1 chopping board**
- **1 sharp knife**
- **1 food processor or blender**
- **measuring spoons**
- **1 mixing bowl**
- **1 mixing spoon**
- **1 freezerproof container with a lid**
- **1 rubber spatula**

1. **Clear** your counter of clutter and **set out** all the equipment you need.
2. **Peel**, **stone** and **chop** the nectarines.
3. **Put** half the raspberries and half the nectarines in a food processor or blender and **process** until smooth.
4. **Stir** the fruit purée and the rest of the fruit into the icing sugar and Greek yogurt in a mixing bowl, then **transfer** to a freezerproof container, cover and **freeze** for 1 hour. **Stir** well, then **cover** and **return** to the freezer and **freeze** until solid.
5. **Serve** the frozen yogurt in scoops, as you would ice cream. It will keep for up to 1 month in the freezer.

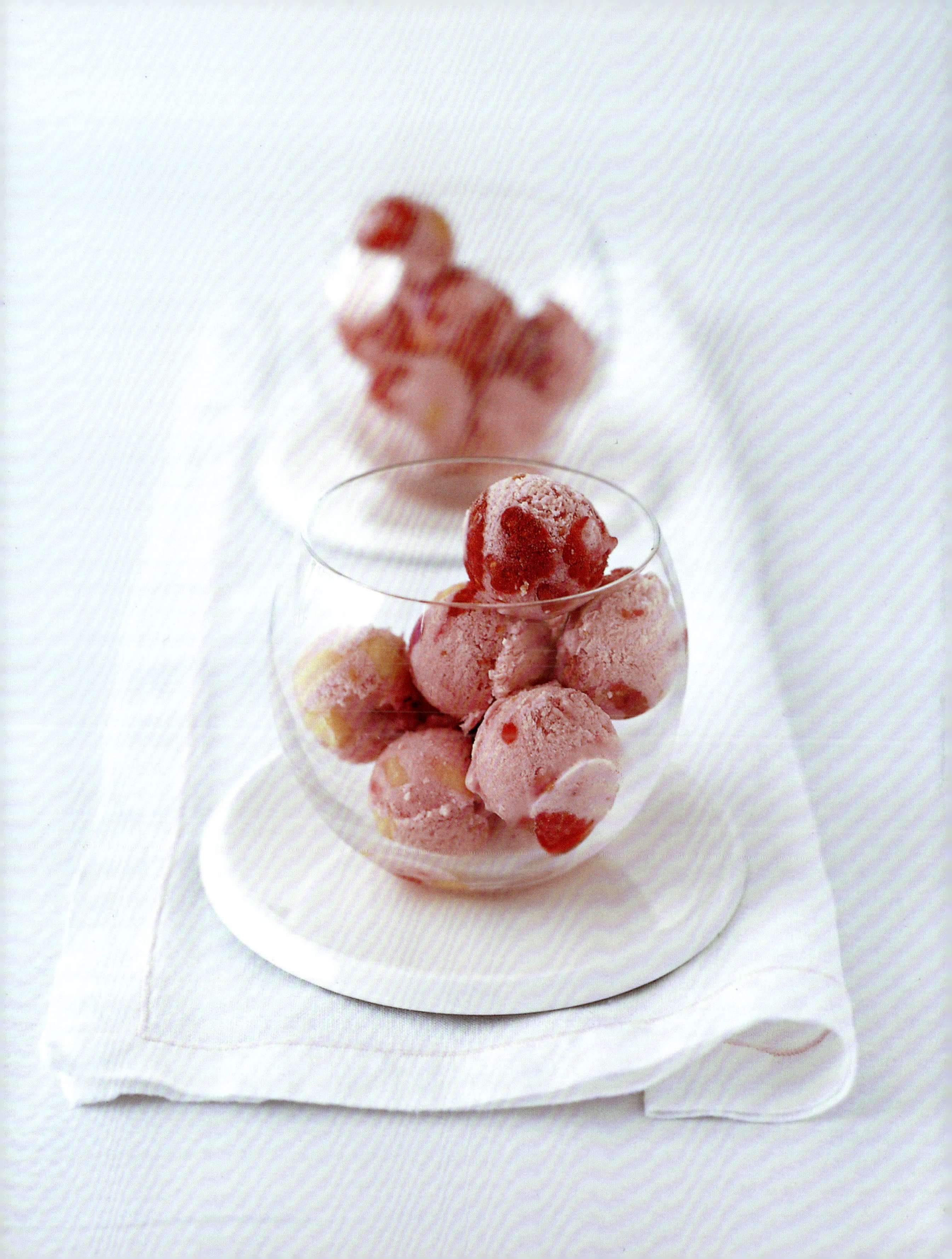

References & Further Reading

American Psychiatric Association: Diagnostic and Statistical Manual of Mental Disorders, Fifth Edition, Text Revision. Washington, DC, American Psychiatric Association, 2022.

Fleming JP, McCauley E, Rodriguez S, O'Connor S and Harsh JR (2021) Effects of ADHD pharmacotherapy on BMI trajectories: A longitudinal study of children and adolescents, Journal of Child Psychology and Psychiatry, 62(12), pp. 1483–1492. (accessed: 12 September 2025).

Grajek M, Krupa-Kotara K, Białek-Dratwa A, Sobczyk K, Grot M, Kowalski O, Staśkiewicz W. Nutrition and mental health: A review of current knowledge about the impact of diet on mental health. Front Nutr. 2022 Aug 22;9:943998. doi: 10.3389/fnut.2022.943998. PMID: 36071944; PMCID: PMC9441951.

Lange KW, Lange K, Nakamura Y, Reißmann A. Nutrition in the management of ADHD: A review of recent research (2023) Current Nutrition Reports [Internet]. Jul 28;12(3):383–94. (accessed 08 August 2025)

McKechnie, D., O'Nions, E., Dunsmuir, S., & Petersen, I., 2023. Attention-deficit hyperactivity disorder diagnoses and prescriptions in UK primary care, 2000–2018: population-based cohort study. *BJPsych Open*, 9.

National Institute for Health and Care Excellence (NICE), 2018. *Attention deficit hyperactivity disorder: diagnosis and management* (Guideline NG87). London: NICE.

Popit, S., Serod, K., Locatelli, I., & Stuhec, M., 2024. Prevalence of attention-deficit hyperactivity disorder (ADHD): systematic review and meta-analysis. *European Psychiatry*, 67.

Other Resources

Books

ADHD an A–Z: Figuring it Out Step by Step by Leanne Maskell (Jessica Kingsley Publishers, 2022)

The Pocket Guide to Neurodiversity by Daniel Aherne (Jessica Kingsley Publishers, 2023)

Unmasked: The Ultimate Guide to ADHD, Autism and Neurodivergence by Ellie Middleton (Penguin Life, 2023)

ADHD Organizations

UK

ADHD UK
adhduk.co.uk

ADDISS (ADHD Information Services)
addiss.co.uk

ADHDadultUK
adhdadult.uk

USA

Children and Adults with Attention-Deficit/Hyperactivity Disorder
chadd.org

Canada

Centre for ADHD Awareness Canada
caddac.ca

Australia

ADHD Australia
adhdaustralia.org.au

New Zealand

ADHD New Zealand
adhd.org.nz

Worldwide

The Attention Deficit Disorder Association
add.org

Find a Dietitian

If you are based in the UK, the British Dietetic Association (BDA) represents the dietetic workforce and offers a directory of freelance dietitians:
bda.uk.com/find-a-dietitian.html

Jacqueline Galanty is a Registered Dietitian and Associate Nutritionist:
nutritionalclinic.co.uk

In the US, the Academy of Nutrition and Dietetics offers a directory of credentialed nutrition and dietetics practitioners:
eatright.org/find-a-nutrition-expert

Eating Disorders

Beat Eating Disorders is a registered charity in the UK that partners with the NHS to provide services for people struggling with eating disorders:
beateatingdisorders.org.uk

Glossary of UK/US Terms

UK	US
Baking paper	Baking parchment
Beetroot	Beet
Bicarbonate of soda	Baking soda
Butter beans	Lima beans
Chickpeas	Garbanzo beans
Coriander (fresh)	Cilantro
Cream, single/double	Cream, light/heavy
Desiccated coconut	Shredded coconut
Dried chilli flakes	Crushed red pepper flakes
Electric whisk	Electric beaters
Flaked almonds	Slivered almonds
Foil	Aluminum foil
Frying pan	Skillet
Grated	Shredded
Grill	Broil
Ground almonds	Almond meal
Jug	Pitcher
Kitchen paper	Paper towel
Minced beef	Ground beef
Mixed spice	Pie spice mix
Natural yogurt	Plain yogurt
Pepper (red)	Bell pepper
Plain dark chocolate	Semi-sweet chocolate
Plain flour	All-purpose flour
Prawns	Shrimp
Rapeseed oil	Canola oil
Rocket	Arugula
Spring onion	Scallion
Stock	Broth
Sugar, caster/icing	Sugar, superfine/ confectioners'
Tomato purée	Tomato paste

Index

About the Author

Jacqueline Galanty is a HCPC-registered dietitian and Associate Nutritionist with experience in both the NHS and private practice. She specialises in working alongside people with neurodivergence and mental health challenges, including ADHD, autism and anxiety.

www.nutritionalclinic.co.uk

Acknowledgements

With special thanks to all my clients and everyone at Octopus who shared their experiences, insights and feedback in the process of making this book.

Photography Credits

iStock: Syuzanna Guseynova 11; Octopus Publishing Group: Craig Robertson 123, 171, David Munns 161, Ian Wallace 43, 133, Lis Parsons 49, 63, 65, 71, 75, 83, 91, 103, 107, 111, 127, 131, 135, 141, 163, 167, 173, 197, 199, 217, Stephen Conroy 53, 79, 89, 169, 201, Will Heap 67, 73, 129, 181, 213, William Lingwood 77, 185, William Reavell 61, 153, 155, 165, William Shaw 45, 47, 55, 57, 59, 81, 87, 93, 95, 99, 101, 105, 109, 115, 117, 119, 121, 125, 137, 139, 145, 147, 149, 151, 157, 159, 175, 177, 179, 187, 189, 191, 193, 203, 207, 211.